ANTI INFLAMMATORY DIET:

This Book Includes:
Anti Inflammatory Diet for Beginners and
Diet Cookbook
Start a Healthy Eating Routine, Improve Your Eating
Habits and Your Immune System with Tasty Recipes.

RIHANNA SMITH

THIS BOOK INCLUDES:

BOOK 1:

ANTI INFLAMMATORY DIET FOR BEGINNERS

All you Need to Know About the Anti-Inflammatory Diet to Heal the Immune System and Prevent Arthritis. Improve your Eating Routine with Healthy Meal Prep Recipes

BOOK 2:

ANTI INFLAMMATORY DIET COOKBOOK

The Book of Easy, Delicious and Tasty Recipes for Beginners, for Establishing New Eating Habits Based on Good Meals and Delicious Recipes

ANTI INFLAMMATORY DIET FOR BEGINNERS

All you Need to Know About the Anti-Inflammatory Diet to Heal the Immune System and Prevent Arthritis. Improve your Eating Routine with Healthy Meal Prep Recipes

RIHANNA SMITH

TABLE OF CONTENTS

ANTI INFLAMMATORY DIET FOR BEGINNERS

Introduction

To better understand the significance of the anti-inflammatory diet, it is important to research the history and fundamentals behind it. In doing this, we can shine a better light on the whole phenomenon. As you will see, it is not a new fad that just gained popularity out of nowhere. A bunch of celebrities did not just start promoting it and now suddenly, it has taken over the world. Never do something just because it is popular. That being said, this particular diet has been popular for a long time. The diet predates modern times and modern medicine. We will touch on the history here so we can better understand the fundamentals. Understanding our history makes it easier to understand our present.

The origins of the anti-inflammatory diet date back to some of the original healers in the world and throughout history. Many of these healers worked with natural herbs, foods, teas, and other holistic remedies to assist the body with its own healing process. Much of these practices are still performed by various people around the world. Without having access to modern, manufactured medications, these natural healers had to make do with what they had. What they did have was an abundance of natural ingredients at their disposal to use for healing or preventing certain ailments. While there may not have been a lot of scientific research to back up many of their claims, much anecdotal evidence suggested that they were on to something. Much of what people discover of the past helped people learn more during the present. While the advent of modern medicines should be held up with pride, it is important to give credit to natural remedies that helped heal people for centuries. Much of it was related to the food people ate.

In more modern times, the anti-inflammatory diet really began getting more mainstream attention from the medical community in the 1970s. Around this time, researchers found that naturally occurring proteins found in our body were a major cause of tissue injury. Before this time, it was believed to be pathogens from outside of the body. This new finding of substances in our own body damaging our own tissues was a big breakthrough for the researchers of this time. They began realizing that our own bodies cells can do just as much, if not more damage than outside sources. Our body literally has the ability to destroy itself. Remember earlier how we spoke of misguided inflammation? This is essentially substances in our own body attacking itself and its own internal tissues, like these proteins, were discovered to do. This was a huge breakthrough for the medical sciences and the makings of an anti-inflammatory diet. Once they discovered this breakthrough, they could better understand how to fix it.

Then in the 1980s, further evidence suggested that various proteins in our bodies were either beneficial or injurious to our bodies' tissues. One of the newly named proteins of this time were called cytokines, which were produced by the immune system. The release of these proteins during the inflammatory process was seen to cause damaging results after the effects of chronic disease. Researchers also began using C-reactive protein, which is a marker of inflammation circulating the

More advanced research found that people with higher levels of C-reactive proteins also had higher levels of heart disease. With much of the research indicating these results, a growing consensus to this day is that inflammation plays a very significant role in the pathogenesis of chronic illnesses like heart disease, lung disease, stroke, diabetes, kidney disease, and even some cancers. For this reason, many medical practitioners and nutrition experts are promoting certain anti-inflammatory diets with foods that will reduce the amount of inflammation in our bodies. This reduced inflammation will result in decreasing or even preventing more chronic illnesses. The anti-inflammatory diet is becoming more prominent as the push to prevent illness rather than cure it is taking off. People are realizing once more that it is better to prevent a catastrophe than deal with its aftermath. The promotion of a proper anti-inflammatory diet coupled with other major lifestyle changes can work wonders for aiding in chronic illnesses.

While we will never discredit the advances of modern medicine, we also want to pay homage to the healers and practitioners of the past. Without the work they did, we would not have made the modern-day strides to continue and advance health and medicine. We also cannot deny that techniques of the past were essential in improving health and we certainly should not avoid these practitioners' contributions for what we have today. Without there knowledge and discoveries, we could not have advanced as much as we have. If it worked for them in the past, then it can work for us today. Modern medicine is needed to deal with some of the advanced medical problems we have today. However, with proper diet and lifestyle, we can prevent those problems from occurring in the first place. Both theories and practices can coexist.

Ancient Greek physician, Hippocrates, who is often considered the Father of Medicine, was one of the first to understand the impact of environment, diet, and lifestyle on human health. Before this, people just related it to external sources like Gods or demons. Hippocrates approach to medicine is far removed from today's medical practices. Modern-day medicine is believed to take a more curative and diagnostic approach, while with Hippocrates, it was focused more on patients care and a good prognosis. Basically, preventative care. Both schools of thought existed in Hippocrates' day, the other one sharing more similarities with the medical practices of today.

Even though much of Hippocrates principles are outdated in ways, his approach can still be heralded as well. With the advent of advanced techniques, we can cure illnesses that were death sentences in years past. It is amazing how far we have come with medical science and we will continue to do so as the years go by. However, our focus with the anti-inflammatory diet somewhat plays off of the teachings of Hippocrates and his beliefs of lifestyle, environment, and diet impacting our health. While at times, extreme measures and advanced medicine is needed, to deny something like diet and lifestyle not having an effect on health is irresponsible.

Let's consider this for a second: remember our two stories from earlier about Tommy and Bobby? Tommy did not use preventative approaches to fix his health. Now, he needs to rely on more advanced medicine to fix his ailments. We applaud the fact that these advanced techniques are available to save Tommy's life. However, we also acknowledge that if Tommy made several lifestyle changes earlier, he may not have needed these more aggressive therapies. With Bobby, he made the changes in his diet early, and for that reason, his health is much better off. We contend that it is better to prevent a heart attack than cure one after the fact.

In summary, the diet in some form has existed for centuries around the world. With further research and determination of the pathogenesis of several diseases, the benefits of the diet's effect on chronic illness are undeniable. We realize that we went more in-depth than we needed to in discussing the science behind inflammatory disease. However, understanding the illness gives us a better understanding of the cure. The anti-inflammatory diet exists also in various forms around the world and we will discuss this further when we get into traveling with the anti-inflammatory diet. There is no one-size-fits-all plan when it comes to this diet and that is what makes it great. Anyone can find food that they love within the parameters of the diet.

What Is Anti Inflammatory Diet

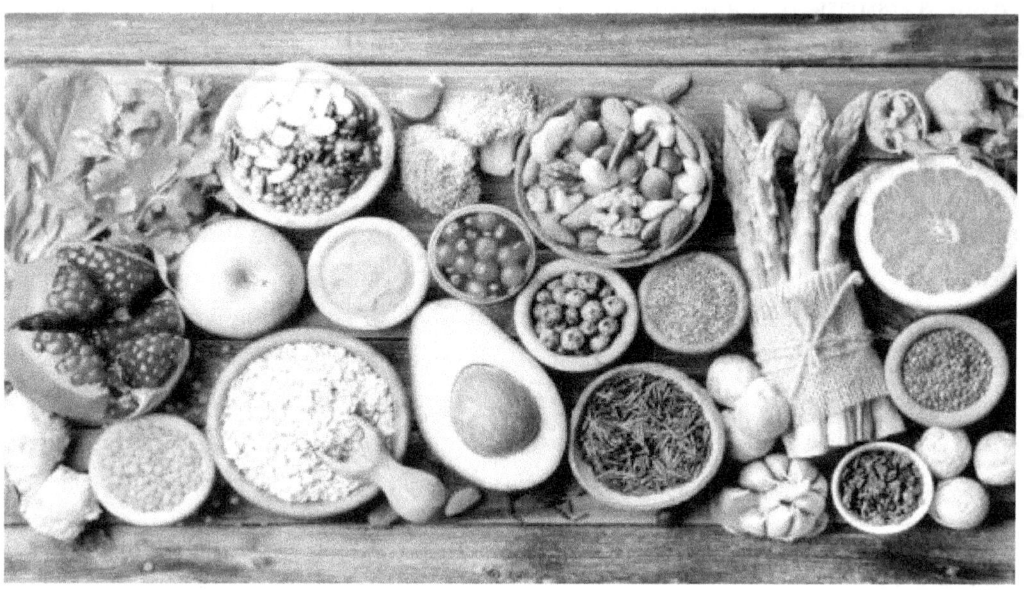

The first step in understanding the need for an anti-inflammatory diet is understanding exactly what inflammation is. The natural response that your body makes when it detects that a harmful invader or a foreign object has invaded its parameters is inflammation. When you become ill or injure yourself in some way, the body will send white blood cells and healing fluids to the sick or injured area in an attempt to eliminate the illness or injury. The natural process of healing begins with inflammation, which should be left alone whenever it is possible to do so. You will first experience irritation. This appears as a fever, stomach ache, or redness or swelling at the site of an injury. You are born with the ability to fight inflammation. Your body can also develop the ability to fight certain inflammations, like the ones caused by a virus or a vaccination.

The body feels two types of inflammation, and they are known as acute or chronic. Acute inflammation is what you feel when you have a cut somewhere on your body, a sore throat, a toothache, or a sprained ankle. It concentrates on the area that needs physical assistance and goes away when the crisis is averted. When your body is first alerted to the presence of inflammation, it is by the cytokines, chemicals that are released by the tissues that have been damaged. The cytokines tell the body's immune system that there is an injury present.

Cytokines are also released when the cause of the inflammation is a chronic reason and not an acute reason. Chronic inflammation is inflammation that occurs over a long time period or comes and goes constantly. Chronic inflammation will have long-lasting effects on your entire body. It is sometimes also called low-grade persistent inflammation because it creates a low level of steady inflammation in the blood, tissues, and muscles in your body. Chronic, systemic inflammation can cause you to develop several different chronic illnesses. Even though these levels of inflammation are low, at least in the beginning, they are enough to trigger an immediate response from your immune system. The white blood cells and other chemicals that your body produces during inflammation will perceive an internal threat and will rush to the inflamed area to protect it. When your white blood cells don't find an obvious cause for the inflammation, they can begin attacking healthy cells, tissue, or internal organs. Chronic inflammation is known to cause several life-threatening illnesses such as cancer, heart disease, and diseases of the circulatory system.

Some inflammation is a natural part of life. Body parts will wear out over time, and you will feel the effects of inflammation when they do. But people who are overweight or eat too many refined foods will suffer more from inflammation than those who carry a normal body weight or eat more of an anti-inflammatory diet. The food that you put into your body will make you feel good, or it will make you feel the effects of inflammation.

The anti-inflammatory diet is not exactly a set dietary plan, as many diets are. When you are following an anti-inflammatory diet, you will base your meals on foods that are known to fight inflammation as well as removing foods from your diet that are known to cause inflammation. You should think of the anti-inflammatory diet as a lifestyle more than you think of it as a diet. It is a particular way of eating that will eliminate or minimize harmful inflammation in your body. Your diet will revolve around veggies and fruits. You will also learn to choose complex carbs over simple carbs, limit your consumption of dairy and red meat, and completely stay away from all processed foods. You will look for fish and veggies that are abundant in their supply of omega-3s, fatty acids that are good for you, and you will limit your intake of inflammation-causing omega-6 fatty acids that you will find in processed foods, commercial salad dressings, mayonnaise, vegetable oil, and corn oil. Certain foods will cause inflammation in the body faster than other foods will. Here are some of the biggest dietary offenders:

Processed Foods

Any food that is processed, even partially, falls into this category. A good example of a partially processed food would be a dinner that comes in a box where you cook the pasta and then add the cheese to the cooked pasta. Snack cakes, chips, and candy are fully processed foods. This list also includes microwave meals, ready-made meals, processed meats, pastries, bread, cold cereal, pre-made dinners, and any fast food.

Transfats and Saturated Fats

Hydrogenated oil causes inflammation because it is full of trans fats, those chemicals that make the fat solid. Trans fats not only cause inflammation on their own, but they also cause inflammation by lowering your good cholesterol and raising your bad cholesterol. You will find hydrogenated oils in ready-made baked goods like pie crusts, cookies, crackers, cakes, and sweet rolls. You will also find them in fried food, margarine, potato chips, refrigerator dough, coffee creamer, and vegetable shortening. Saturated fats in foods can also add to or cause inflammation. They can also lead to cholesterol level imbalances and heart disease. Saturated fat is found in the skin of poultry, milk, pork, butter, palm oil, coconut oil, cheese, and red meat.

Alternative or Artificial Sweeteners

These are often used by people who are trying to cut their dependence on real sugar since sugar is known to cause inflammation. But alternative and artificial sweeteners also have the same effects on the body as real sugar does, so they are no better for your body than real sugar is. These sweeteners can cause muscle aches, vomiting, fatigue, headache, abdominal pain, joint pain, nausea, mood swings, skin rashes, and insomnia. The only exception to this is saccharin since it does not seem to have the same negative effects on the body as other artificial or alternative sweeteners do.

Carbohydrates

Not all carbs will lead to an increase in inflammation in your body, but some will. There are many different foods that are in the group of foods known as carbs. A carb is a food compound that contains starch, sugar, and cellulose. You will find carbs in grains, fruits, veggies, and milk, and these are the good carbs. The bad carbs are found in cakes, cookies, sweet rolls, muffins, and bread. You can divide carbs into two categories that are called complex and simple. The complex carbs are the grains, veggies, and fruits that do not cause inflammation in your body. The processed foods and bakery goods fall into the group that is known as simple carbs, and they are the ones that cause inflammation.

When you begin consuming a diet that is based on anti-inflammatory foods, then you will notice that the inflammation that is already present in your body will begin to lessen. This way of eating will also help to prevent the formation of future inflammation. Anyone can reap the benefits of the anti-inflammatory diet. You will be eating the good types of foods that your body needs to allow it to prevent inflammation from forming and relieving the inflammation that has already formed. The anti-inflammatory diet is based on the types of healthy foods that your body needs to heal itself. Your diet will be based on fruits and veggies, plant-based proteins like beans and nuts, whole grains, fatty fish, and plenty of herbs and spices to add flavor to your food.

Fruits and Veggies

All veggies and fruits are full of nutrients that will help you to eliminate or prevent inflammation, like minerals, vitamins, and phytonutrients. These compounds are the antioxidants that your body needs to fight the oxidants in your body. Oxidants are also known as free radicals, cells that are formed during the process of metabolism that breaks free and causes inflammation in your body while they work to destroy healthy cells. Free radicals will put you at a greater risk of developing chronic illnesses. One type of antioxidant is found in the chemicals that give fruits and veggies their deep, rich color, like the greens, reds, and oranges found in a diet based on fruits and veggies. Another type of antioxidant is known as anthocyanins which also help to fight free radicals in your body and are found in the deep-colored foods, the ones that are purple and blue. And all fruits and veggies are full of fiber that will feed the good bacteria in your gut and by keeping your digestive tract clean.

Seafood, Fish, and Meat

Poultry and meat are high in their content of omega-6 fatty acids, which are the fats that cause inflammation. While it is not necessary to completely eliminate those foods, it will be better for your health if you can limit them, or even eliminate them completely. Most seafood and fatty fish are high in omega-3 fatty acids, which will eliminate inflammation while they are preventing their development.

Whole Grains

A grain needs to have all three parts intact to be able to be called a whole grain. On a piece of grain, the outer layer is the bran, the fiber of the grain. The middle layer is the starchy part, and the little seed inside is the part that holds the vitamins and the healthy fats. When grains are refined the healthy bran and the vitamin-filled seed are discarded; the only part that is left is the starchy middle part. That part holds the least amount of nutrition and causes the most inflammation when it is consumed without the other parts. Whole grains also have a certain amount of fiber that will feed the good bacteria that lives in your gut and works to keep your digestive tract clean. Every day at least half of the food you consume should be whole grains of some sort.

Legumes

Legumes are full of phytonutrients that work as antioxidants in your body, and they are rich in B-vitamins, minerals, and fiber. All of the legumes are good for you. They will help to reduce the inflammation in your body as well as decreasing your appetite and aiding in the reduction of your risk of developing diabetes, heart disease, and obesity.

Tea, Coffee, and Dark Chocolate

All of these are made from plants that are rich in phytonutrients, and all have caffeine that is known to reduce inflammation in the body. It is best to keep your intake of coffee to less than three cups every day. Tea is a better drink for the body and should be consumed often. When you eat dark chocolate, make sure it is seventy percent chocolate or higher.

Oils and Nuts

Seeds, nuts, and oils are good for preventing or reducing inflammation in the body, but they are high in fat, which in itself can cause inflammation, so their consumption should be limited to two or three tablespoons each day.

Herbs and Spices

There are so many different flavors that can be achieved by the use of herbs and spices. And many of these ingredients are known to be medicinal in nature, so they will also prevent the formation of inflammation or help to reduce it.

You can easily develop an eating plan that is based on anti-inflammatory foods. These foods will help to reduce the inflammation that is already present in your body and will help to prevent more inflammation from forming.

Benefits of the Anti-Inflammatory Diet

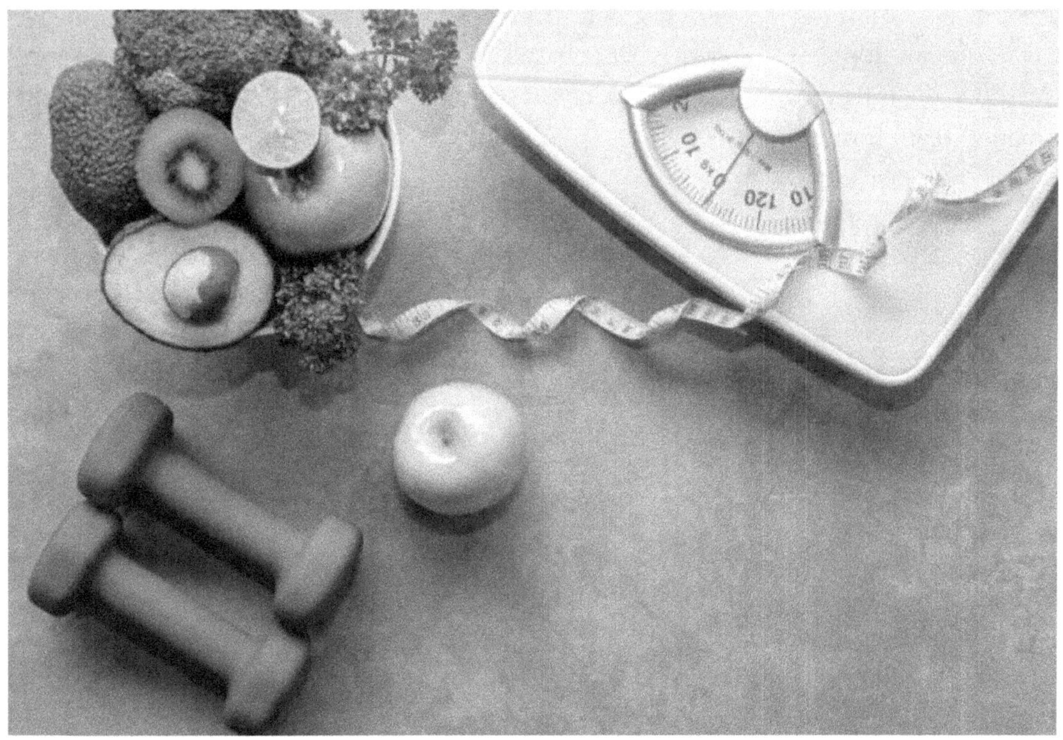

The anti-inflammatory diet has a lot of health benefits. Surprisingly, it has similar benefits to the top leading diet out there. Make sure you read them, allowing you to understand how this diet can help you in the long run. One thing we want you to keep in mind would be that many users might notice different results from this diet. Many users claim benefits that are not even listed here since they are not so common. The anti-inflammatory diet is truly a surprise when it comes to delivering the results; this diet works very differently on everyone else.

Make sure that you understand that you will see benefits that are not common, most likely. However, you will see the basic benefits of this diet, regardless of who you are. I would also like to point out that these benefits are from personal experience only, even though some have been backed up by science that does not mean all of them are. You see, the health and fitness industry is so personal that getting an accurate understanding of what a certain diet could do is very much impossible. All we can do is understand the studies which have been done by scientist and try and relate it to us, which is all we can do in terms of getting to understand what the anti-inflammatory diet can offer us in terms of health benefits. We will list out all of the most common benefits associated with this diet, but please keep in mind that you might see different results from this diet and that it can be quite different from what you expected. None the less, this is one diet you have to test out for yourself.

Weight-Loss

As you know, there are many ways to lose weight. However, one of the most popular methods being used to lose weight is the anti-inflammatory diet, and there is a good reason behind it. Many people do not know this, but the anti-inflammatory diet is perhaps the best way for someone to lose "body fat" instead of "body-weight." When following most diets, followers tend to lose a ton of weight, but most of the time, it is muscle and water weight they are getting rid of.

On the other hand, the anti-inflammatory diet makes you lose more body fat. Here is how it works, when you are eating right healthy foods for a prolonged period, you have burned out all your glycogen stores as your caloric intake drops. Which makes the body hit your reserves, and that, of course, is your body fat. You will be burning more body fat instead of muscle mass or glycogen, which makes it ideal for people looking to lose weight. Also, as you know, proper diet plays a huge role in affecting your hormones. Your insulin will flatline, and your growth hormone will go up, this will prime your body to burn body fat instead and will do so in a healthy manner.

Increased Longevity

There have been many studies showings that the anti-inflammatory diet can boost endurance. As you might know by now that anti-inflammatory diet can help you with cell rejuvenation or also known as autophagy, this process enables you to get rid of the old and weak cells and replace it with newer, stronger ones. This process has shown to increase longevity and overall well-being, which is one of the reasons why the anti-inflammatory diet can help you live a longer life. Moreover, some studies are showing that reducing calories in animals by 30% to 40% has shown to increase their lifespan. However, there is no study done on humans claiming such. Nonetheless, some studies are suggesting that monkeys that ate less food but more on the anti-inflammatory side lived longer. However, there was another study indicating that it wasn't the case on 25-year-old long research done by another party.

Although there is no actual study backing these claims up, it does show that people who ate less had fewer risks of diseases, which could lead to longevity. Which is excellent news when looking at it from that angle, there is a lot of disease prevention that comes with the anti-inflammatory diet. However, the main thing to remember would be the fact that an anti-inflammatory diet helps with autophagy, which enables you to rejuvenate cells, which makes it very evident that the anti-inflammatory diet can help you with longevity and overall well-being, which is a great thing to consider.

Prevent Diseases

There are many diseases present in today's day and age, and it very common to meet someone suffering from one. This means we need to figure out a way to reduce the risk of diseases for overall health and well-being. The anti-inflammatory diet has shown to lower the risk of many diseases, and we will be discussing all the disorders the anti-inflammatory diet can help get rid of. One of the many conditions anti-inflammatory diet could help manage would be Alzheimer's and Parkinson's.

As you know, the anti-inflammatory diet helps boost brain health and to lower the risk of neurologic diseases. Some studies are showing that the anti-inflammatory diet can help reduce the risk of depression, even though some people might not consider this a condition, it is still a significant issue in our society. The anti-inflammatory diet has also shown to reduce cholesterol. A 2010 study on overweight women found that the anti-inflammatory diet improved hosts of health complications, including cholesterol levels (LDL) and blood pressure, which is also known as the silent killer.

The anti-inflammatory diet also helps with reducing type 2 diabetes, and there was one study done on men, which showed that anti-inflammatory helped them stop insulin treatment. Although we do not recommend you try this if you have type 2 diabetes, that goes to show you the power of the diet and insulin resistance.

Nonetheless, many studies are suggesting that the anti-inflammatory diet can lower the risk of diabetes. Another devastating disease in which an anti-inflammatory diet helps getting rid of would be cancer. As you know, the anti-inflammatory diet enables you to have a less hospitable environment for the cancer cells, which makes this diet an excellent idea for people who are looking to reduce this risk.

In regards to a healthier life, the anti-inflammatory diet has also shown to reduce the risk of obesity. One study done on obese women suggested that an anti-inflammatory diet reduced the risk of obesity in women, which makes sense as it helps you lose and manage body weight.

These facts about the anti-inflammatory diet show you how the anti-inflammatory diet can help you get free of many diseases, and some have been backed up with detailed studies, whereas others are still being researched.

Nonetheless, you can't say that about other diets out there. The anti-inflammatory diet will help you to get rid of many things and prevent you from further having any diseases. There is no better way of getting rid of illness or problems without the use of modern medicine, and this diet is so powerful that it will also boost your immune system, which will help you avoid small issues like the common flu. All in all, there are many rejuvenating properties that come along with the anti-inflammatory diet, so do not overlook it and keep all the positives in mind before you look at the negatives.

Reduce Stress and Inflammation

The anti-inflammatory diet has shown a significant reduction in inflammation. As you know, inflammation causes many chronic diseases such as Alzheimer's, dementia, obesity, diabetes, and much more. Now, there are many ways that the anti-inflammatory diet helps you get rid of inflammation. The first one being autophagy, as you know, anti-inflammatory diet helps you with cell rejuvenation cleans up itself by eating out the old self and rejuvenating them with the newer, stronger ones. If your body does not regenerate itself with more new cells, the older ones that have stayed for an extended period can cause inflammation.

Now that we've talked about many ways. An anti-inflammatory diet enables you to reduce inflammation; let us talk about how the anti-inflammatory diet can help you get rid of stress. You see, inflammation and stress go hand in hand. If you have high levels of inflammation, chances are your stress levels are going to be higher. This means that if you lower your inflammation, you will reduce your stress levels, and as you know, this diet helps with better brain function. An anti-inflammatory diet enables you to send better signals to your brain, which would equal a better functioning brain.

When your mind is functioning at its absolute peak, your levels of stress dropdown. Better brain function will also help you get rid of any stress you might be having and will give you overall better health can help you reduce weight. Overall, the health benefits you get from the anti-inflammatory diet will help you get rid of your stress or at least lower it. This means, even if you are not facing any stress-related issues, the anti-inflammatory diet will help you have a better functioning brain and also help you get rid of any mental fog or stress you might be dealing with. With that in mind, always make sure you consult a physician if you are noticing much more stress than you can handle, as it can be something severe and not fixable by the anti-inflammatory diet.

Boost Immune System

There is a reason why having a healthy immune system is fundamental, as it will help you get less sick and be more "immune" to disease. The anti-inflammatory diet has shown to increase the immune system, so we will talk about how it boosts the immune system. There was a study done on stem cells when it comes down to a diet individual; more specifically, they took a look at how the stem cells rejuvenated.

The study concluded that anti-inflammatory diet depleted white blood cells, which is precisely what we want so our body can produce better and more efficient cells, which lead to more production of stem cells and lesser of white cells. Once you start to get rid of your old white blood cells, you will begin to produce new ones, which will overall help you recover faster. This study also found that there was a reduced amount of protein kinase A (PKA), which allows the stem cells to regenerate. If you have a lower amount of (PKA), this means that it will enable the cells to turn on the regeneration mode, which will allow them to create new cells.

As you know, the anti-inflammatory diet has shown to reduce insulin levels, which is a great thing for someone looking to boost their immune system. There was a study done showing that high amounts of insulin levels, prevented "T" cells from doing its job effectively. The "T" cells are here to suppress inflammation, and to fight off illness, "T" cells are most of the time responsible for getting rid of toxins, which cause disease and inflammation. When your insulin levels are high, "T" cells are not performing at their highest potential, which causes our immune system to drop down.

When you are diet, there isn't a requirement for insulin spikes, which lets our body help the "T" cells work at a higher level and, overall, boosting our immune system. Since you aren't eating foods that will spike your insulin a crazy amount, this will give your digestive system and organs a break. When you eat a big meal, around 70% of the blood and energy goes to your stomach to digest it. This means when you are on a diet, you give your body a chance to recover. Everything is healing when you are on the anti-inflammatory diet, which includes the digestive system. Meaning, your gut will be working a lot more effectively once you have given it some time to heal.

As you know, digestion plays a significant role in both our mental health and immune system, about 60% of our immune system is in our colon, which means when you are the diet, you are recovering your whole body and overall boosting your immune system. You will be doing yourself an excellent service if you can manage to boost your immune system, and with all the backed-up science showing how anti-inflammatory diet can help you promote your immune system and reduce many other health problems, there is no reason not to start the anti-inflammatory diet as soon as possible.

More Energy and Muscle Mass Increased

Even if your goal isn't to put on more muscle, it is still good to have more muscle mass as it helps you with many things. However, the main thing having higher amounts of muscle mass helps you with would be a fat loss; having a higher muscle mass will help you burn more fat since it increases your metabolic rate. Do not worry, and you do not have to look like a bodybuilder for that to happen; nonetheless, it is essential to have the right amount of muscle mass, especially for women.

The anti-inflammatory diet has shown to increase and preserve muscle mass, so let us talk about how that happens. There was a study done between two groups of men, one followed an 80/20 diet method, and the other followed a healthy eating pattern. Both groups followed the same workout but a different diet, one group which supported the 80/20 diet, which we will talk about later in this book, they noticed after eight weeks was, both the groups gained and preserved the same amount of muscle, but the group who were following the anti-inflammatory diet lost more fat.

This shows that the anti-inflammatory diet not only helped followers gain muscle and preserve it, but it also helped them lose fat simultaneously. The main reason behind that is growth hormone, as you know, the anti-inflammatory diet has shown to increase growth hormone in our bodies. What growth hormone mainly does, it allows a lot less muscle breakdown and to burn more fat, which is one of the main reasons why the anti-inflammatory diet is so beneficial for building and preserving muscle mass.

Another great benefit of the anti-inflammatory diet, as you know, is higher energy levels, and there is a reason behind it. Many people know how it feels to have a sugar crash, you feel tired and lethargic, and the culprit behind it is insulin. When insulin is spiked up, your energy level goes down as this gives your brain a signal to relax. When you are an anti-inflammatory diet, there are no insulin spikes throughout the day, which provides you with more energy.

Another reason why you have more energy when you are diet is that your body goes into a fight or flight response and since your body is eating food it was intended to eat in the first place, and our body produces more adrenaline throughout the day, which gives you more energy as you go along. Just be aware, at the beginning of your diet journey, you might feel less energized.

The reason behind it is because your body is still getting used to these changes, but after a week or two, you should start to notice more energy. Use the power to get more work done at work and gym. In my opinion, and this is the most significant benefit which comes along with the anti-inflammatory diet. More energy makes you feel a lot better when you are looking towards making it through those long days.

These are all the main benefits that come along when you start the diet, and the benefits genuinely outweigh all the negatives which might happen. These benefits can be life-changing to most people, lowering the risk of diseases and increasing longevity it's a fantastic thing to have. anti-inflammatory diet provides you with that and then some.

Foods to Eat

Inflammation friendly foods follow the one principle of thought mentioned before, "The farther away it is from its natural state, the more inflammatory it's inclined to be".

It's also important to recognize your own tolerances and in-tolerances when it comes to choosing your fresh foods. For example, some experts believe people with arthritis should avoid the nightshade family of vegetables and other experts suggest not to avoid that class of vegetables at all. It can get a bit confusing when they are all talking about combating inflammation, so let me make it simple.

Tomatoes, white potatoes, peppers, and eggplants are all classified as nightshade vegetables. Some people report they have less joint pain when they don't eat these veggies, but research has not substantiated this. These vegetables do contain, for example, lycopene and vitamin C that help restrain inflammation as in the case of tomatoes.

Here is a good rule to follow. We are all unique, and we all tolerate and have in-tolerances to different foods and chemicals, each of us has our own unique food sensitivities and some even have food allergies uniquely their own. Whenever you find you have these sensitivities, it only makes sense that you leave them out of your diet.

Sensitivities show up after we eat something that makes us feel uncomfortable or even unwell.

Simply cut them from your diet going forward. If you know you have a sensitivity to something in the list below, merely substitute it for something similar on the list that does not affect you in the same way, maybe it is from the nightshade family, but it has never bothered you in the past, this would still be a good choice.

A study conducted with women suffering from rheumatoid arthritis reported they experienced fewer joint pains and more flexibility when they awoke after staying on a Mediterranean diet for at least 2 months. They were also given a cooking class on Mediterranean-style foods to help them stay on the diet.

Omega-3 fatty acids - Foods commonly found in foods from our Mediterranean friends are heavy in omega-3. These fats have been clinically shown to lower inflammation. Fatty fish are where omega-3s are located in plenty, but other good sources as well that I have listed below:

- Salmon

- Tuna

- Sardines

- anchovies

- Mackerel

- Halibut, trout, and herring

- Walnuts - Persian walnuts

- Flaxseeds and flaxseed oil

- Pumpkin seeds

- Chia seeds

- Extra virgin olive oil helps to keep the anti-inflammatory properties of the food you are cooking. It also has antibacterial properties and is a good inflammation fighter.

Meats - Avoid meats that have not been grass fed. Organic is a good choice as most of those animals are grass fed. Red meat can be high in fat so choose leaner portions if you find yourself craving a good steak.

Red meats are not on our list below, but some people find it hard to give up, especially in the beginning. Processed meats or meats that have been smoked, cured or treated with chemicals are also on the unfriendly inflammation list.

Proteins are what we're after in our meat choices, we need them to build cells and our immune system uses them in spades for the creation of antibodies. We can find good protein sources in vegetables too and a good idea to mix it up to find the right amounts. Not including vegetables in the mix would result in excessive fat intake, and we would miss out on the rich nutrients provided by vegetable proteins.

- Lean skinless chicken, turkey or wild game - organic is preferred as it's free of chemical processes. 2 times a week is a good rule of thumb.

- Atlantic cod, wild salmon, rainbow trout, tilapia

- Canned tuna and sardines

- Scallops, shrimp, and squid

Proteins found in Vegetables, grains, beans, legumes, and nuts - these can be packed with proteins as much as meats and come without the unnecessary fat content.

Here are some power packed protein sources:

•	Quinoa - our bodies need 22 amino acids to make protein and quinoa has every single one of them and is also gluten-free.

•	Nuts and seeds - such as almonds, cashews, and sunflower seed. Don't worry about the high fat in nuts - it's mostly the good kind. Here are some other tasty nuts:

•	Pistachios

•	Pine Nuts

•	Pumpkin seeds

•	Walnuts

•	Beans and legumes - a powerful source of protein, these are often called "natures perfect foods". If you think they are too high in fat, think again, they contain less than 1% fat per serving and again, it's the good kind of fat.

•	Edamame leads the way in protein with 68 grams of protein per 1 cup

•	Great northern beans

•	Lentils

•	White beans

•	Yellow beans

•	Pinto beans

•	Black beans

•	Cannellini beans

•	Red beans

•	Kidney beans

•	Grains - avoid processed grains and opt for whole grains like brown rice (brown basmati rice is my personal favorite; it has a nice nutty flavor) quinoa and millet. Whole grains help reduce the inflammatory hormone homocysteine in our bodies.

•	Vegetables - green and green leafy vegetables are brimming with A, C, and K. These vitamins protect us from of the dangers of the free kind, and their high content of calcium keeps our bones strong.

•	Broccoli

•	Green leafy spring lettuce

•	Brussel sprouts

•	Kale

•	Swiss chard

•	Bok choy

•	Spinach

•	Tomatoes - contain lycopene and vitamin C that help restrain inflammation

•	Chili peppers - contain capsaicin, natural pain and inflammation fighter

•	Fresh vegetables - living foods for our live bodies

More.......

Citrus fruits - boost our immune system which can stave off inflammatory diseases like rheumatoid arthritis. They contain vitamin C which also assists our immune system.

The berries listed below from the red berry family; contain powerful antioxidants that hold down inflammation:

•	Oranges

•	grapefruits

•	limes

•	Cherries

•	Blueberries

•	Raspberries

•	Strawberries

•	Blackberries

Other good foods for an anti-inflammatory diet:

- Coconut

- olives

- Avocados

- Cocoa

- Mushrooms - all kinds, eat lots of them

- Grapes

I am sure you are beginning to see a pattern developing between good anti-inflammatory fighting foods and foods that contribute to the buildup of inflammation.

I've tried to put together a comprehensive list of foods you can start to incorporate into your anti-inflammatory diet routine, but each time my research seems to have reached an end other good sources suddenly show themselves, which leads me to believe that I probably have just touched the surface. I highly recommend if you find yourself wondering if a certain food item you are considering has anti inflammatory benefits or one that you should avoid, do a search on the internet or at your local library.

I often find, if I have a question and not sure if something is good for the anti-inflammation front, I can find good medical research or opinions that will help me to form my own assumptions and then I can try it out and see if it helps me individually.

It's a good idea to talk with your personal physician if you take medications. Some food and spices can have unwanted side effects if taken with certain medications.

Spices and Herbs That Add an Anti-Inflammatory Punch

Spices and herbs can be fun to experiment with in cooking meals, but you can also use them in your smoothie preparation, and soups are always a hit when you add herbs and spices, so be sure to always have on hand anti-inflammatory spices and herbs. This is one quick way you can make sure you add a punch to your anti-inflammatory diet. Here are some good ones to put on your shopping list:

- Paprika - a tasty spice that is produced in sweet or smoky flavors. Constructed from different types of bell and chili peppers that are roasted and ground. No wonder it's so tasty! Loaded with capsaicin, which is a natural inflammatory opponent and antioxidant. It protects our bodies from cell damage. It's great on meat and vegetables alike - chicken, steak, grilled eggplant, in salad dressings, you get the picture.

•	Turmeric - has an exotic ancient history, it has permeated the Middle East and Southeastern Asian food and medical cultures for centuries, for good reason, it's a power-packed spice. Just a tablespoon of turmeric harbors a gram of protein, twenty-nine calories, two grams of fiber and six grams of carbohydrates, minerals such as manganese, phosphorus, and potassium, curcumin. Used to treat inflammation and a myriad of other ailments in ancient civilizations. Today you can find it by itself or in curry or yellow mustard. WebMD recommends trying it as a tea or in a smoothie before you opt in for the over-the-counter painkillers.

•	Cinnamon - Recent lab studies have found that cinnamon reduces inflammation, fights bacteria and acts as an antioxidant, but is still unproven in the effects on people. Still, a flavorful choice to sprinkle on toast, add to your morning coffee (a great way to get your cinnamon without adding sugar). Pretty delicious when you make cocoa, cinnamon and banana smoothie or soak cinnamon bark sticks in apple tea with honey.

•	Ginger - also used for hundreds of years to treat gastrointestinal problems and rheumatoid arthritis pain. It's no surprise that it has anti-inflammatory properties. You can use ginger in a variety of ways from smoothies, soups, and teas to cooking in fish and stir-fry dishes. I have a sampling of each of these in the recipe section of this book.

•	Garlic - is an anti-inflammatory superstar (onions too), but for the greatest benefits use it raw versus a powder form. Garlic inhibits the production of cytokines. Cytokines are responsible for calling for an inflammatory response.

•	Curry - this spice pumps up its anti-inflammatory package. It has both turmeric and curcumin, powerful inflammation fighters. Curry is also deeply flavorful, so if you find yourself with bland food on your plate, add a little curry and see what happens.

•	Cardamom - found in pumpkin spice mixes and is sweet and pungent. Indian dishes use this spice and lab studies show it may help fight inflammation and soothe an upset stomach.

•	Cumin - is noticeably used in Indian and Spanish dishes. A good spice to add to an anti-inflammatory diet due to its weight loss benefits. A recent study of 88 overweight women who included a teaspoon of cumin daily in conjunction with a low carb diet lost more body fat than those on the same diet without adding the cumin.

•	Cocoa - is a fun spice, we often associate it with chocolate so our eyes and ears light up at the thought of such a treat, but it can also make us feel we are cheating on any diet we are participating in. Yet, cocoa has many health perks too, one is anti-inflammatory properties and the other is antioxidants. Cocoa has flavanols which are responsible for the anti-inflammatory effects, and they keep the cells that line your arteries healthy.

•	Rosemary - doesn't have the anti-inflammatory superpowers that ginger has, it still curbs inflammation. It also is a powerful antioxidant and has high levels of calcium, iron, and vitamin B6.

•	Clove–Studies are still uncertain yet, but there are indications they may possess anti-inflammatory qualities. Used to care for stomach problems, nausea, and inflammations found in the mouth and throat, so chances are it will add to our anti-inflammation fighting regime.

•	Cayenne -and other hot chili peppers have recognized inflammatory benefits. An age-old capsaicin is known for its anti-inflammation fighting qualities.

•	Green Tea - an herb made from tea leaves, is a rich source of polyphenols, and The Arthritis Foundation recognizes polyphenols are strong anti-inflammatories.

Add these spices to boost your anti-inflammatory regime and help your body overthrow inflammation headed your way.

Food to Avoid

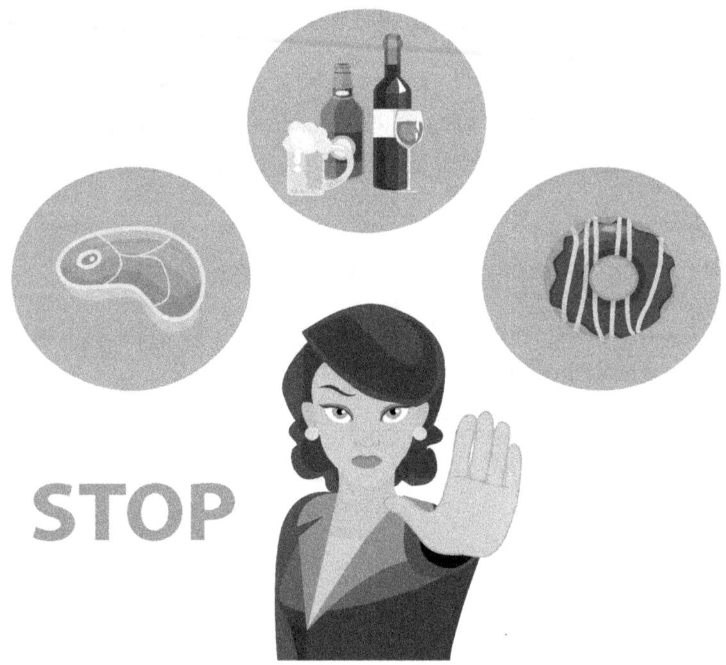

Our eating habits and the foods that we eat may cause inflammation. One of the ways that you can kick start your way into the anti-inflammatory diet is to avoid eating inflammation causing foods.

These foods can be placed in six different categories:

1.   High Fructose and Sugary Foods

2.   Vegetable Oils (Includes Seed Oils)

3.   Excess Alcohol

4.   Processed Meat

5.   Refined Carbs

6.   Artificial Trans Fats

Let's go over the details of each of these items and why they can cause inflammation.

High Fructose and Sugary Foods

On the top of our list of foods that you should avoid are sugary foods and foods that contain a lot of fructose. There are two main culprits in our day to day diet that contribute to inflammation.

The first one is high fructose corn syrup and the other one is table sugar. These are the two main types of sugar that is very common in our modern diet. According to one study, these added sugars actually cause a lot of damage to the body.

According to another study, it is possible to develop breast cancer with a high sucrose diet. Sucrose is another form of sugar. It is also suggested that eating sugary foods can prevent or block the anti-inflammatory effects of omega-3 fatty acids.

Now, fructose and all the other types of sugars that you find naturally in all our foods are not bad or evil per se. They're actually good—they give the body its needed energy. What's bad is taking in too much—which can happen really quickly.

Just drink a large can of Coke and you would have ingested all the sugar that your body needs in one week in just one sitting. But do you stop with one can of soda? Some people drink three sodas or more each day.

High fructose intake has been linked to chronic diseases like cancer, fatty liver disease, diabetes, insulin resistance, obesity, and chronic kidney disease.

Foods that usually have high levels of added sugar include the following:

- Certain types of cereals

- Sweet pastries

- Doughnuts

- Cookies

- Cakes

- Soft drinks

- Chocolates

- Candy

- Fruit juices (sweetened ones)

- Any sugar sweetened drinks

Vegetable Oils (Includes Seed Oils)

The average consumption of veggie oils and seed oils has increased in the 20th century by as much as 130%. Experts see it as a contributor to the growing number of health problems caused by inflammation. Researchers believe that increased consumption of these oils causes inflammation.

These oils contain a lot of omega-6 fatty acids. Even though they are necessary to the human body, they actually increase inflammation when there is more omega-6 compared to omega-3 in the body.

Note that vegetable oils are used in cooking and are ingredients in a lot of processed foods as well. Reduce your intake of veggie oils and seed oils so as to prevent the onset or to reduce inflammation in the body.

Excess Alcohol

It can be argued that moderate alcohol consumption does have some health benefits. That means your occasional couple of drinks every now and then isn't really that bad. However, taking in more alcohol than usual will cause serious health problems including inflammation.

People who have a heavy drinking problem may have the tendency to accumulate bacterial toxins in the body—a condition known as leaky gut syndrome. This condition can lead to organ damage and widespread inflammation.

Processed Meat

Processed meat includes beef jerky, smoked meat, ham, bacon, and sausages. They taste great and some people have made them staples on the dining table. However, studies suggest that these foods have been associated with increased risk of a variety of diseases including colon cancer, stomach cancer, diabetes, and heart disease.

The most common illness connected with processed meat consumption is colon cancer. Researchers suggest that this might be due to the fact that these meats contain a large amount of advanced glycation end products or AGEs. AGEs are formed when meat is combined with other substances and then exposed to high temperatures.

Studies confirm that AGEs cause inflammation in the body. Note that there are many factors that contribute to the development of colon cancer. However, research suggests that the biggest contributing factor is probably the consumption of processed meat and the inflammation that comes with it.

Refined Carbs

Not all carbs are created alike. Some are nice to have and there are those that can be a good part of your diet. The ones that are nice to have aren't exactly necessary—and I'm referring to refined carbohydrates.

Note that not every kind of carb is problematic. You see, since ancient times man has been consuming carbs. It's a fact, but our ancestors ate unprocessed carbs and it contained a lot of fiber, which is good for the body.

What has changed in the last hundred or so years is that we have introduced refined carbs. The idea behind using refined carbs is that the refining process lengthens the shelf life of the carbs that we usually produce.

However, in the process of refinement, the fiber and all the other essential nutrients get stripped off. What we have left are the refined carbohydrates. Sure they have really longer shelf life but they can cause a lot of inflammation, according to studies.

Remember that fiber promotes blood sugar control and it basically makes you feel full. That is why you don't crave for more food when you just had a high fiber diet. Fiber also feeds the good bacteria in your gut, which helps to maintain your overall health.

Why are refined carbs bad for you? Research suggests that the bacteria that are responsible for inflammation in your gut feed off refined carbs. When inflammation becomes chronic due to years of poor eating choices, then inflammation in the gut will become problematic.

Refined carbs also have a high glycemic index (GI) compared to unprocessed carbs. When food has a rather high GI, it can raise your blood sugar a lot faster. Studies suggest that eating too much food that have a high GI may cause chronic obstructive pulmonary disease

Artificial Trans Fats

The unhealthiest fats on the planet are none other than artificial trans fats. These are foods that have partially hydrogenated ingredients. What that means is that hydrogen is added to unsaturated fats. Unsaturated fats usually have a liquid form. By adding hydrogen to them they become more solid which makes them more stable.

If you check the label on certain food packages, these are the ingredients that have the words "partially hydrogenated" and then followed by the ingredient name. Most margarine brands have trans fats. They are added to extend the shelf life.

Note however that there are natural trans fats as well. These are the fats that are produced in the body and they can also be found in meat as well as in dairy products. It is the artificial trans fats that studies point to that increases our risk for diseases and also cause of inflammation.

Artificial trans fats also reduce the amount of good cholesterol (HDL) in the body. Studies also show that they also impair the endothelial cells lining our arteries which increase our risk for heart disease.

Foods that are usually cooked with artificial trans fats include certain types of pastries, cookies, packaged cakes, vegetable shortening, margarine, microwave popcorn, French fries, and other types of fast food.

30 Days Meal Plan

Day	Breakfast	Lunch	Snacks	Dinner	Dessert
1	Easy Almond Zucchini Bowl	Salmon and Sweet Potato Mix	Simple Yet Effective Vegan Truffle	Tasty Turkey Baked Balls	Chickpeas Salad
2	Blueberry and Cashew Mix	Cod and Tarragon Sauce	Guilt and Dairy "Free" Chocolate Pudding	Chicken, Corn & Spinach Sauté	Quinoa and Beans
3	Tomato and Olive Salad	Shrimp and Mango Mix	A Very Subtle Cherry Crisp	Sprouts & Slices In Wheat Wrap	Cucumber and Green Onions Salad
4	Sweet Potato Hash	Orange Chicken Salad	Delicious Pumpkin Pie "Spicy" Pastries	Feta-Filled & Tomato-Topped Turkey Burger Bites	Barley and Kale
5	Avocado Omelet	Brown Rice and Chicken Mix	Cool And Warm Oven Roasted Plums	Simply Sautéed Flaky Fillet	Herbed Mango Mix
6	Coconut Porridge	Greek Chicken Breasts	Apples With A Fire Within	Spicy Sautéed Chinese Chicken	Cabbage Slaw
7	Broccoli and Squash Mix	Easy Chicken and Potato Mix	Awesome and Crunchy Muffins	Tasty Thai Chicken in Crisp Cups	Cucumber with Apples Salad
8	Greens and Berries Mix	Paprika Chicken Mix	The Cherry Beet Delight	Zesty Zucchini & Chicken In Classic Santa Fe Stir-Fry	Parsley Avocado Mix
9	Veggie and Eggs	Veggie Lunch Salad	Green Delight	Crispy Cheese-Crusted Fish Fillet	Endives and Broccoli

10	Coconut Pear Bowl	Grilled Eggplant Lunch Salad	Easy Chia Seed Pumpkin Pudding	Ambrosial Avocado & Salmon Salad in Lemon-Dressed Layers	Arugula Salad
11	Blackberry and Strawberry Salad	Eggplant and Avocado Lunch Mix	The Mediterranean Fruit Granita	Sautéed Shrimp Jambalaya Jumble	Chickpeas Salad
12	Breakfast Kale Frittata	Eggplant and Egg Mix	Guilt Free Lemon And Rosemary Drink	Toasted Tilapia Topped with Panko & Pecans	Quinoa and Beans
13	Cranberry Granola Bars	Eggplant and Egg Mix	Strawberry and Rhubarb Smoothie	Tortilla Tostadas with Peppered Potato & Kingly Kale	Cucumber and Green Onions Salad
14	Spinach and Berry Smoothie	Veggie Soup	Vanilla Hemp Drink	Turkey Tomato Sweet Potato Stuffed Peppers	Barley and Kale
15	Zucchini Breakfast Salad	Shrimp Soup	Yogurt and Kale Smoothie	Baked Buffalo Cauliflower Chunks	Herbed Mango Mix
16	Early Morning Pesto Eggs	Chicken and Veggies	Spiced Kale Chips	Cool Garbanzo and Spinach Beans	Cabbage Slaw
17	Shrimp and Egg Medley	Hidden Valley Chicken Drummies	Vegetable Nuggets	Lemony Garlic Shrimp	Cucumber with Apples Salad
18	Old Fashioned Breakfast Oatmeal	Lemon-Parsley Chicken Breast	Cabbage Pineapple Slaw	Coconut and Hazelnut Chilled Glass	Parsley Avocado Mix
19	Barley Porridge	Lemony Mussels	Turmeric Muffins	Coriander Greens with Zucchini Sauté!	Endives and Broccoli

20	Hearty Banana Oatmeal	Hot Tuna Steak	Coffee Protein Bars	Walnuts and Asparagus Delight	Arugula Salad
21	Pumpkin And Cinnamon Porridge Meal	Marinated Fish Steaks	Cauliflower Popcorn	Butternut Squash with Lentils	Chickpeas Salad
22	Scrambled Turkey Eggs	Lime Pork and Green Beans	Spiced Pumpkin Seeds	Buckwheat Noodle Pad Thai	Quinoa and Beans
23	Cinnamon Baked Apple Chips	Pork with Lemongrass	Curry Roasted Chickpeas	White Beans and Olive Stuffed Zucchinis	Cucumber and Green Onions Salad
24	Herb and Avocado Omelet	Pork with Olives	Coconut Oats Balls	Buckwheat and Sweet Potatoes	Barley and Kale
25	The Blueberry and Avocado Medley	Pork Chops with Tomato Salsa	Seasoned Coconut Flakes	Zucchini Patties	Herbed Mango Mix
26	Lovely Pumpkin Oats	Cabbage Orange Salad with Citrusy Vinaigrette	Turmeric Bars	Shrimp Mix	Cabbage Slaw
27	Cool Cinnamon And Pear Oatmeal	Lemon Buttery Shrimp Rice	Anti-Inflammatory Turmeric Gummies	Spinach and Lentils Stew	Cucumber with Apples Salad
28	Healthy Zucchini Stir Fry	Valencia Salad	Ginger Spiced Mixed Nuts	Sweet Potato Mix	Parsley Avocado Mix
29	Simple Blueberry Oatmeal	Tenderloin Stir Fry with Red And Green Grapes	Spicy Tuna Rolls	Pea Stew	Endives and Broccoli
30	Morning Smoothie Bowl	Aioli with Eggs	Veggie Burrito	Green Beans Stew	Arugula Salad

Breakfast Recipe

1. Easy Almond Zucchini Bowl

Preparation time: 10 minutes

Cooking time: 15 minutes

Servings: 2

Ingredients:

1 cup egg whites, whisked

1½ tablespoons ground flaxseed

1 cup almond milk, unsweetened

1 banana, peeled and mashed

1 small zucchini, grated

½ teaspoon ground cinnamon

Directions:

In a small pan, combine the milk with the egg whites, flaxseed, banana, zucchini and cinnamon powder. Bring to a simmer, mixing constantly, over medium heat. Cook for 15 minutes, divide into bowls and serve for breakfast.

Enjoy!

Nutrition:

Calories: 201 Cal Fat: 6 g

Fiber: 9 g Carbs: 14 g

Protein: 6 g

2. Blueberry and Cashew Mix

Preparation time: 10 minutes

Cooking time: 12 minutes

Servings: 2

Ingredients:

2 bananas, peeled and sliced

¼ cup cashews

¼ cup blueberries

1 tablespoon almond butter

1/3 cup coconut flakes, unsweetened

1 cup coconut milk, unsweetened

Directions:

In a small pot, mix the berries with the coconut flakes, milk, cashews, almond butter and bananas. Mix together and bring to a simmer over medium heat. Cook for 12 minutes, divide into bowls and serve for breakfast.

Enjoy!

Nutrition:

Calories: 370 Cal Fat: 23 g

Fiber: 6 g Carbs: 40 g

Protein: 8 g

3. Tomato and Olive Salad

Preparation time: 10 minutes

Cooking time: 0 minutes

Servings: 4

Ingredients:

2 cups baby spinach, torn

2 cups cherry tomatoes, halved

4 tablespoons chopped red onion

1 cup chopped cucumber

1 cup kalamata olives, pitted and sliced

1 tablespoon chopped dill

3 tablespoons lemon juice

A pinch of salt and black pepper

2 tablespoons olive oil

Directions:

In a salad bowl, toss the spinach with the tomatoes, onion, cucumber, olives, dill, lemon juice, salt, pepper and oil. Serve for breakfast.

Enjoy!

Nutrition:

Calories: 171 Cal Fat: 2 g

Fiber: 5 g Carbs: 11 g

Protein: 5 g

4. Sweet Potato Hash

Preparation time: 10 minutes

Cooking time: 15 minutes

Servings: 4

Ingredients:

1 sweet potato, peeled and cubed

1 celery root, peeled and cubed

1 cup coconut milk

2 tablespoons olive oil

1 small yellow onion, chopped

1 teaspoon smoked paprika

4 garlic cloves, minced

2 tablespoons parsley, chopped

A pinch of salt and black pepper

Directions:

Heat up a pan with the oil over medium-high heat. Add the celery root and the sweet potato, toss and cook for 5 minutes. Add the onion, garlic, salt, pepper, parsley and paprika then toss and cook for 8 minutes more. Add the coconut milk, mix and cook for 1-2 minutes. Divide everything into bowls and serve for breakfast.

Enjoy!

Nutrition:

Calories: 188 Cal Fat: 2 g Fiber: 8 g

Carbs: 10 g Protein: 4 g

5. Avocado Omelet

Preparation time: 10 minutes

Cooking time: 10 minutes

Servings: 2

Ingredients:

4 eggs, whisked

2 avocados, pitted, peeled and cubed

A pinch of salt and black pepper

Juice of ½ lemon

1 tablespoon chopped parsley

1 tablespoon olive oil

Directions:

In a bowl, mix the eggs with the avocados, salt, pepper, lemon juice and parsley. Heat up a pan with the oil over medium-high heat then add the avocado and egg mix, spread into the pan and cook for 4 minutes on each side. Divide between plates and serve for breakfast.

Enjoy!

Nutrition

Calories: 201 Cal

Fat: 2 g

Fiber: 5 g

Carbs: 1 g

Protein: 5 g

6. Coconut Porridge

Preparation time: 10 minutes

Cooking time: 15 minutes

Servings: 2

Ingredients:

2 cups coconut milk, unsweetened

3 tablespoons almond flour

½ cup coconut flakes, unsweetened

2 tablespoons ground flax meal

1 teaspoon vanilla extract

2 teaspoons ground cinnamon

Directions:

In a small pot, mix the coconut milk with the almond flour, coconut flakes, flax meal, vanilla and cinnamon. Stir and bring to a simmer over medium heat for 15 minutes. Divide into bowls and serve for breakfast.

Enjoy!

Nutrition:

Calories: 287 Cal

Fat: 5 g

Fiber: 7 g

Carbs: 13 g

Protein: 5 g

7. Broccoli and Squash Mix

Preparation time: 10 minutes

Cooking time: 15 minutes

Servings: 4

Ingredients:

4 cups spaghetti squash, peeled, cooked and flesh scrapped out

1½ cups broccoli florets

1 tablespoon olive oil

1 cup coconut milk, unsweetened

1 egg, whisked

1 teaspoon garlic powder

A pinch of salt and black pepper

Directions:

Heat up a pan with the oil over medium-high heat, add the spaghetti squash and the broccoli. Stir and cook for 5-6 minutes. Add the garlic powder, salt, pepper, garlic powder and the egg. Stir and cook for 5 minutes more. Add the coconut milk, mix and cook for about 5 minutes more then divide into bowls and serve for breakfast.

Enjoy!

Nutrition:

Calories: 207 Cal Fat: 5 g

Fiber: 8 g Carbs: 1 g

Protein: 7 g

8. Greens and Berries Mix

Preparation time: 10 minutes

Cooking time: 0 minutes

Servings: 2

Ingredients:

½ cup spinach, torn

½ cup kale, torn

1 cup strawberries, halved

1 cup blueberries

1 banana, peeled and chopped

6 mint leaves, chopped

Directions:

In a bowl, mix the spinach with the kale, strawberries, blueberries, banana and mint. Serve for breakfast.

Enjoy!

Nutrition:

Calories: 198 Cal

Fat: 4 g

Fiber: 2 g

Carbs: 8 g

Protein: 6 g

9. Veggie and Eggs

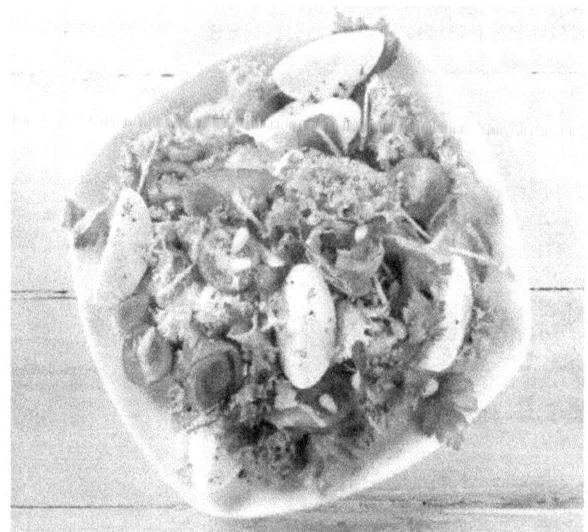

Preparation time: 10 minutes

Cooking time: 15 minutes

Servings: 6

Ingredients: 1 red bell pepper, chopped

4 cherry tomatoes, chopped

3 spring onions, chopped

A handful kale, torn

1 tablespoon olive oil   6 eggs

A pinch of salt and black pepper

A pinch of curry powder

Directions:

Heat up a pan with the oil over medium-high heat, add the onions, stir and cook for 1-2 minutes. Add the bell pepper, the tomatoes, the kale, salt, pepper and the curry powder, stir and cook for 4-5 minutes. Crack the eggs into the pan and mix well. Cook until the eggs are done, divide between plates and serve for breakfast.   Enjoy!

Nutrition: Calories: 106 Cal Fat: 8 g

Fiber:1 g Carbs. 4 gProtein: 7 g

10. Coconut Pear Bowl

Preparation time: 10 minutes

Cooking time: 15 minutes

Servings: 4

Ingredients:

2 cups coconut milk, unsweetened

1/3 cup coconut flakes, unsweetened

½ teaspoon vanilla extract

3 pears, peeled, cored and cubed

Directions:

Put the milk in a small pot, add the coconut, vanilla and pears. Stir and bring to a simmer over medium heat, cook for 15 minutes, divide into bowls and serve.

Enjoy!

Nutrition:

Calories: 172 Cal

Fat: 5 g

Fiber: 7 g

Carbs: 8 g

 Protein: 4 g

11. Blackberry and Strawberry Salad

Preparation time: 5 minutes

Cooking time: 0 minutes

Servings: 1

Ingredients:

¼ cup sliced almonds

¼ cup blackberries

¼ cup strawberries, halved

1 banana, peeled and sliced

A pinch of ground cinnamon

Directions:

In a bowl, mix the blackberries with strawberries, cinnamon, banana and almonds. Serve for breakfast.

Enjoy!

Nutrition:

Calories: 90 Cal

Fat: 3 g

Fiber: 1 g

Carbs: 0

Protein: 5 g

12. Breakfast Kale Frittata

Preparation time: 10 minutes

Cooking time: 30 minutes

Servings: 4

Ingredients:

6 kale stalks, chopped

1 small sweet onion, chopped

1 small broccoli head, florets separated

2 garlic cloves, minced

Salt and black pepper to the taste

4 eggs

1 tablespoon olive oil

Directions:

Heat up a pan with the oil over medium-high heat, add the onion, stir and cook for 4-5 minutes. Add the garlic, broccoli and kale, toss and cook for 5 minutes more. Add the eggs, salt and pepper and mix. Place in the oven and bake at 380 degrees F for 20 minutes. Slice and serve for breakfast.

Enjoy!

Nutrition:

Calories: 214 Cal

Fat: 7 g Fiber: 2 g

Carbs: 12 g Protein: 8 g

13. Cranberry Granola Bars

Preparation time: 2 hours

Cooking time: 0 minutes

Servings: 4

Ingredients:

2 cups walnuts, toasted

1 cup dates, pitted

3 tablespoons water

¾ cup cranberries, dried, no added sugar

2 cups desiccated coconut, unsweetened

Directions:

In your food processor, mix dates with coconut, cranberries, water and walnuts. Pulse really well then spread the mix into a lined baking dish. Press well into the dish and keep in the fridge for 2 hours then cut into bars and serve.

Enjoy!

Nutrition:

Calories: 476 Cal

Fat: 40 g

Fiber: 9 g

Carbs: 33 g

Protein: 6 g

14. Spinach and Berry Smoothie

Preparation time: 10 minutes

Cooking time: 0 minutes

Servings: 2

Ingredients:

1 cup blackberries

1 avocado, pitted, peeled and chopped

1 banana, peeled and roughly chopped

1 cup baby spinach

1 tablespoon hemp seeds

1 cup water

½ cup almond milk, unsweetened

Directions:

In your blender, mix the berries with the avocado, banana, spinach, hemp seeds, water and almond milk. Pulse well, divide into 2 glasses and serve for breakfast.

Enjoy!

Nutrition:

Calories: 160 Cal

Fat: 3 g

Fiber: 4 g

Carbs: 6 g

Protein: 2 g

15. Zucchini Breakfast Salad

Preparation time: 10 minutes

Cooking time: 0 minutes

Servings: 4

Ingredients:

2 zucchinis, spiralized

1 cup beets, baked, peeled and grated

½ bunch kale, chopped

2 tablespoons olive oil

For the tahini sauce:

1 tablespoon maple syrup

Juice of 1 lime

¼ inch fresh ginger, grated

1/3 cup sesame seed paste

Directions:

In a salad bowl, mix the zucchinis with the beets, kale and oil. In another small bowl, whisk the maple syrup with lime juice, ginger and sesame paste. Pour the dressing over the salad, toss and serve it for breakfast.

Enjoy!

Nutrition:

Calories: 183 Cal Fat: 3 g

Fiber: 2 g Carbs: 7 g

Protein: 9 g

16. Early Morning Pesto Eggs

Preparation Time: 5 minutes

Cooking Time: 5 minutes

Servings: 2

Ingredients 2 large whole eggs

1/2 tablespoon almond butter

1/2 tablespoon pesto

1 tablespoon creamed coconut almond milk

Sunflower seeds and pepper as needed

Directions:

Take a bowl and crack open your egg.

Season with a pinch of sunflower seeds and pepper.

Pour eggs into a pan.

Add almond butter and introduce heat.

Cook on low heat and gently add pesto.

Once the egg is cooked and scrambled, remove heat.

Spoon in coconut cream and mix well.

Turn on the heat and cook on LOW for a while until you have a creamy texture.

Serve and enjoy!

Nutrition: Calories: 467 Cal

Fat: 41 g Carbohydrates: 3 g

Protein: 20 g

17. Shrimp and Egg Medley

Preparation Time: 15 minutes

Cooking Time: 0

Servings: 4

Ingredients:

4 hardboiled eggs, peeled and chopped

1-pound cooked shrimp, peeled and deveined, chopped

1 sprig fresh dill, chopped

¼ cup mayonnaise

1 teaspoon Dijon mustard

4 fresh lettuce leaves

Directions:

Take a large serving bowl and add the listed Ingredients (except lettuce)

Stir well

Serve over bet of lettuce leaves

Enjoy!

Nutrition:

Calories: 292 Cal

Fat: 17 g

Carbohydrates: 1.6 g

Protein: 30 g

18. Old Fashioned Breakfast Oatmeal

Preparation Time: 10 minutes

Cooking Time: 5 minutes

Servings: 4

Ingredients:

2 and ½ cups of water

1 cup of old-fashioned oats

1 cup apple, peeled, cored and chopped

3 tablespoons of almond butter

2 tablespoon of palm sugar

½ a teaspoon of cinnamon powder

Directions:

Add water, oats, apple, butter, cinnamon, and sugar to our pot

Toss well and lock the lid

Cook on HIGH pressure for 5 minutes

Release the pressure naturally over 10 minutes

Stir oats and divide into bowls. Enjoy!

Nutrition:

Calories: 191 Cal

Fat: 2 g

Carbohydrates: 9 g

Protein: 5 g

19. Barley Porridge

Preparation Time: 5 minutes

Cooking Time: 25 minutes

Servings: 4

Ingredients:

1 cup barley

1 cup of wheat berries

2 cups unsweetened almond milk

2 cups of water

Toppings such as hazelnuts, honey, berry, etc.

Directions:

Take a medium saucepan and place it over medium-high heat

Place barley, almond milk, wheat berries, water and bring to a boil

Lower down the heat to low and simmer for 25 minutes

Divide amongst serving bowls and top with your desired toppings. Serve and enjoy!

Nutrition:

Calories: 295 Cal

Fat: 8 g

Carbohydrates: 56 g

Protein: 6 g

20. Hearty Banana Oatmeal

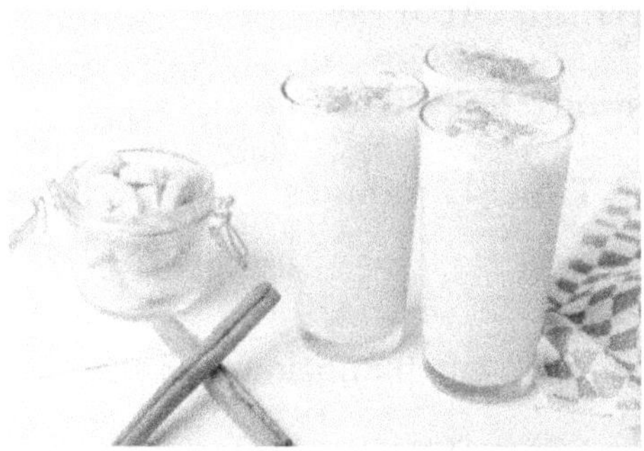

Preparation Time: 10 minutes

Cooking Time: 10 minutes

Servings: 4

Ingredients: 2 cups of water

1 cup steel-cut oats 1 cup of almond milk

¼ cup walnuts, chopped

2 tablespoon of flaxseeds, ground

2 tablespoon of chia seeds

2 bananas, peeled and mashed

1 teaspoon of vanilla extract

1 teaspoon of cinnamon powder

Directions: Add water, oats, almond milk, flaxseed, walnuts, chia seeds, vanilla, bananas, cinnamon to your Pot and give it a nice toss Lock up the lid and cook on HIGH pressure for 10 minutes Release the pressure naturally and open the lid Divide the mix amongst bowls and serve Enjoy!

Nutrition: Calories: 200 Cal Fat: 4 g Carbohydrates: 11 g Protein: 4 g

21. Pumpkin and Cinnamon Porridge Meal

Preparation Time: 10 minutes

Cooking Time: 15 minutes

Servings: 2

Ingredients: ½ cup pumpkin puree

1 cup unsweetened almond/coconut milk

1 cup of water 1 cup uncooked quinoa

1 teaspoon ground cinnamon

2 tablespoon ground flaxseed meal

Juice of 1 lemon

Directions:

Take a pot and place it over medium-high heat

Whisk in water, almond milk and bring the mix to a boil

Stir in quinoa, cinnamon, and pumpkin

Lower heat to low and simmer for 10 minutes until the liquid has been evaporated

Remove heat and stir in flaxseed meal

Transfer porridge to small bowls

Sprinkle lemon juice and add pumpkin seeds on top. Serve and enjoy!

Nutrition: Calories: 245 Cal

Fat: 1 g Carbohydrates: 59 g

Protein: 4 g

22. Scrambled Turkey Eggs

Preparation Time: 15 minutes

Cooking Time: 15 minutes

Servings: 2

Ingredients: 1 tablespoon coconut oil

1 medium red bell pepper, diced

½ medium yellow onion, diced

¼ teaspoon hot pepper sauce

3 large free-range eggs ¼ teaspoon salt

¼ teaspoon black pepper, freshly ground

Directions:

Set a pan to medium-high heat and add coconut oil, let it heat up

Add onions and Sauté

Add turkey and red pepper

Cook until turkey is cooked

Take a bowl and beat eggs, stir in salt and pepper

Pour eggs in the pan with turkey and gently cook and scramble eggs

Top with hot sauce and enjoy!

Nutrition:

Calories: 435 Cal Fat: 30 g

Carbohydrates: 34 g

Protein: 16 g

23. Cinnamon Baked Apple Chips

Preparation Time: 5 minutes

Cooking Time: 2 hours

Servings: 2

Ingredients:

1 teaspoon cinnamon

1-2 apples

Directions:

Preheat your oven to 200 degrees Fahrenheit

Take a sharp knife and slice apples into thin slices

Discard seeds

Line a baking sheet with parchment paper and arrange apples on it

Make sure they do not overlap

Once done, sprinkle cinnamon over apples

Bake in the oven for 1 hour

Flip and bake for an hour more until no longer moist

Serve and enjoy!

Nutrition:

Calories: 147 Cal

Fat: 0

Carbohydrates: 39 g

Protein: 1 g

24. Herb and Avocado Omelet

Preparation Time: 2 minutes

Cooking Time: 10 minutes

Servings: 2

Ingredients:

3 large free-range eggs

½ medium avocado, sliced

½ cup almonds, sliced

Salt and pepper as needed

Directions:

Take a non-stick skillet and place it over medium-high heat

Take a bowl and add eggs, beat the eggs

Pour to the skillet and cook for 1 minute

Lower heat to low and cook for 4 minutes

Top the omelet with almonds and avocado

Sprinkle salt and pepper and serve

Enjoy!

Nutrition:

Calories: 193 Cal

Fat: 15 g

Carbohydrates: 5 g

Protein: 10 g

25. The Blueberry and Avocado Medley

Preparation Time: 5 minutes

Cooking Time: 0

Servings: 4

Ingredients:

1 frozen banana

2 avocados, quartered

2 cups berries

Maple syrup as needed

Directions:

Take your blender and add all Ingredients except maple syrup

Add ice water and blend

Garnish with syrup and pour in smoothie glasses

Enjoy!

Nutrition:

Calories: 250 Cal

Fat: 13 g

Carbohydrates: 40 g

Protein 4 g

26. Lovely Pumpkin Oats

Preparation Time: 5 minutes

Cooking Time: 8 minutes

Servings: 3

Ingredients:

1 cup quick-cooking rolled oats

¾ cup almond milk

½ cup canned pumpkin puree

¼ teaspoon pumpkin pie spice

1 teaspoon ground cinnamon

Directions:

Take a safe microwave bowl and add oats, almond milk, and microwave on high for 1-2 minutes

Add more almond milk if needed to achieve your desired consistency

Cook for 30 seconds more

Stir in pumpkin puree, pumpkin pie spice, ground cinnamon

Heat gently and enjoy!

Nutrition:

Calories: 229 Cal

Fat: 4 g

Carbohydrates: 38 g

Protein:10 g

27. Cool Cinnamon and Pear Oatmeal

Preparation Time: 10 minutes

Cooking Time: 15 minutes

Servings: 2

Ingredients:

3 cups of water

1 cup steel-cut oats

1 tablespoon cinnamon powder

1 cup pear, cored and peeled, cubed

Directions:

Take a pot and add water, oats, cinnamon, pear and toss well

Bring it to simmer over medium heat

Let it cook for 15 minutes, divide amongst the bowl

Enjoy!

Nutrition:

Calories: 171 Cal

Fat: 5 g

Carbohydrates: 11 g

Protein: 6 g

28. Healthy Zucchini Stir Fry

Preparation Time: 10 minutes

Cooking Time: 10 minutes

Servings: 4

Ingredients:

2 tablespoons of heaping olive oil

1 whole medium-sized onion, sliced thinly

2 whole medium-sized zucchini, cut up into thin sized strips

2 heaping tablespoons of teriyaki flavored sauce, low sodium

1 whole tablespoon of coconut aminos

1 whole tablespoon of a sesame seed, toasted

Ground pepper (black) as much as needed

Directions:

Take a skillet and place it over medium level heat. Add onions, and stir cook for 5 minutes

Add your zucchini and stir cook for 1 minute more. Gently add the sauces alongside the sesame seeds

Cook for 5 minutes more until the zucchini are soft

Finally, add in pepper and enjoy!

Nutrition: Calories: 110 Cal

Fat: 9 g Carbohydrates: 8 g

Protein: 3 g

29. Simple Blueberry Oatmeal

Preparation Time: 10 minutes

Cooking Time: 8 hours

Servings: 4

Ingredients:

1 cup blueberries

1 cup steel-cut oats

1 cup of coconut milk

2 tablespoons agave nectar

½ teaspoon vanilla extract

Coconut flakes, garnish

Directions:

Grease Slow Cooker with cooking spray

Add oats, milk, nectar, blueberries, and vanilla

Toss well

Place lid and cook on LOW for 8 hours

Divide between serving bowls and serve

Enjoy!

Nutrition:

Calories: 202 Cal

Fat: 6 g

Carbohydrates: 12 g

Protein: 6 g

30. Morning Smoothie Bowl

Preparation Time: 10 minutes

Cooking Time: 0

Servings: 2

Ingredients:

2 cups baby spinach leaves

1 cup coconut almond milk

¼ cup low fat cream

2 tablespoons flaxseed oil

2 tablespoons chia seeds

2 tablespoons walnuts, roughly chopped

A handful of fresh berries

Directions:

Add spinach leaves, coconut almond milk, cream and flaxseed oil to a blender

Blitz until smooth

Pour smoothie into serving bowls

Sprinkle chia seeds, berries, walnuts on top

Serve and enjoy!

Nutrition:

Calories: 380 Cal

Fat: 36 g

Carbohydrates: 12 g

Protein: 5 g

Lunch Recipes

31. Salmon and Sweet Potato Mix

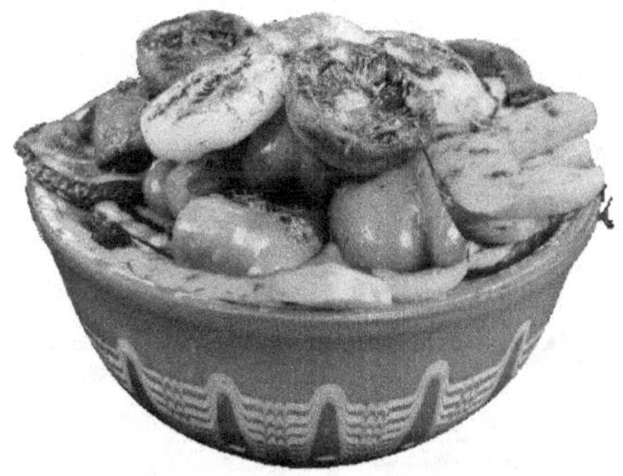

Preparation times: 10 minutes

Cooking time: 0 minutes

Servings: 4

Ingredients: 1 tablespoon olive oil

1½ pounds sweet potatoes, baked and cubed

4 ounces smoked salmon, chopped

1 tablespoon chopped chives

2 teaspoons horseradish

¼ cup coconut cream

Salt and black pepper to the taste

Directions:

In a bowl, whisk together the coconut cream with salt, pepper, horseradish and chives. Add salmon and potatoes, toss to coat and serve right away. Enjoy!

Nutrition: Calories: 233 Cal Fat: 6 g

Fiber: 5 g Carbs: 37 g Protein :9 g

32. Cod and Tarragon Sauce

Preparation time: 10 minutes

Cooking time: 15 minutes

Servings: 4

Ingredients: 2 tablespoons mustard

4 medium cod fillets, skinless and boneless

1 tablespoon chopped tarragon

1 tablespoon capers, drained

4 tablespoons olive oil+ 1 teaspoon

Salt and black pepper to the taste

2 cups lettuce leaves, torn

1 small red onion, sliced

1 small cucumber, sliced

2 tablespoons lemon juice   2 tablespoons water

Directions: In a bowl, mix mustard with 2 tablespoons olive oil, tarragon, capers and water, whisk well and set aside. Heat up a pan with 1 teaspoon oil over medium-high heat. Season fish with salt and pepper to the taste then add to pan and cook for 6 minutes on each side. In a separate bowl, mix cucumber with onion, lettuce, lemon juice, 2 tablespoons olive oil, salt and pepper to the taste. Arrange the cod between plates, drizzle the tarragon sauce all over and serve with the cucumber salad on the side.   Enjoy!

Nutrition: Calories 261 Cal Fat 8, Fiber 1 g

Carbs 8 g Protein 14 g

33. Shrimp and Mango Mix

Preparation time: 10 minutes

Cooking time: 0 minutes

Servings: 5

Ingredients:

2 tablespoons Dijon mustard

3 tablespoons white wine vinegar

6 tablespoons avocado mayonnaise

4 cucumbers, peeled and cubed

1 mango, peeled and cubed

3 tablespoons chopped dill

1-pound shrimp, cooked, peeled and deveined

A pinch of salt and black pepper

Directions:

In a salad bowl, mix the cucumbers with the mango, shrimp, dill, salt and pepper and toss.

Add the mustard, vinegar and mayonnaise and mix well then serve.

Enjoy!

Nutrition:

Calories: 174 Cal

Fat: 3 g

Fiber: 2 g

Carbs: 4 g

34. Orange Chicken Salad

Preparation time: 10 minutes

Cooking time: 30 minutes

Servings: 4

Ingredients:

1 whole chicken, cut into medium pieces

4 scallions, chopped

2 celery ribs, chopped

1 cup chopped mandarin orange

¼ cup avocado mayonnaise

½ cup coconut cream

1 cup chopped cashews, toasted

A pinch of salt and black pepper

Directions:

Put chicken pieces in a pot and add water to cover. Add a pinch of salt then bring to a boil over medium heat and cook for 25 minutes. Transfer to a cutting board, discard bones, shred meat and put in a bowl. Add celery, orange pieces, cashews, scallion, salt, pepper, mayo and the coconut cream, toss to coat and serve.

Enjoy!

Nutrition:

Calories: 210 g

Fat: 3 g

Fiber: 3 g

Carbs: 16 g

Protein: 18 g

35. Brown Rice and Chicken Mix

Preparation time: 10 minutes

Cooking time: 10 minutes

Servings: 4

Ingredients:

1½ cups brown rice, cooked

1½ tablespoons coconut sugar

1 cup chicken stock

2 tablespoon coconut aminos

4 ounces chicken breast boneless, skinless and cut into small pieces

1 egg

2 egg whites

2 scallions, chopped

Directions:

Put stock in a pot, heat up over medium-low heat and add coconut aminos and sugar, stir, bring to a boil, add the chicken and toss. In a bowl, mix the egg with egg whites, whisk well then add over the chicken mix. Sprinkle the scallions on top and cook for 3 minutes without stirring. Divide the rice into 4 bowls, add the chicken mix on top and serve.

Enjoy!

Nutrition:

Calories: 231 g

Fat: 11 g

Fiber: 7 g

Carbs: 8 g

Protein: 9 g

36. Greek Chicken Breasts

Preparation time: 10 minutes

Cooking time: 30 minutes

Servings: 6

Ingredients:

6 chicken breast halves, skinless and boneless

2 teaspoons olive oil

½ cup vegetable stock

1 tablespoon chopped basil

2 teaspoons chopped thyme

½ cup chopped yellow onion

3 garlic cloves, minced

½ cup kalamata olives, pitted and sliced

¼ cup chopped parsley

3 cups chopped tomatoes

Directions:

Heat up a pan with the oil over medium heat, add chicken and cook for 6 minutes on each side. Transfer cooked chicken to a plate. Heat up the same pan used for the chicken over medium heat, add garlic, stir and cook for 1 minute. Add onion, tomatoes and the stock then stir and bring to a simmer. Cook for 10 minutes. Add basil, thyme and the chicken, mix and cook for 12 minutes. Add parsley, olives, salt and pepper, toss, divide between plates and serve.

Enjoy!

Nutrition: Calories: 221 Cal

Fat: 2 g Fiber: 4 gCarbs: 7 g

Protein: 8 g

37. Easy Chicken and Potato Mix

Preparation time: 10 minutes

Cooking time: 50 minutes

Servings: 4

Ingredients:

1 tablespoon olive oil

4 teaspoons garlic, minced

A pinch of salt and black pepper

¼ teaspoon dried thyme

12 small red potatoes, halved

Cooking spray

2 pounds chicken breast, skinless, boneless and cubed

1 cup sliced red onion

¾ cup vegetable stock

½ cup pepperoncini peppers, chopped

2 cups chopped tomato

¼ cup kalamata olives, pitted and halved

2 tablespoons chopped basil

14 ounces canned artichokes, drained and chopped

Directions:

In a baking dish, mix potatoes with 2 teaspoons garlic, olive oil, thyme, salt and pepper. Bake in the oven at 400 degrees F for 30 minutes. Heat up a pot over medium-high heat, grease with cooking spray, add chicken, season with salt and black pepper and cook for 5 minutes on each side then transfer to a plate. Heat up the pot again over medium heat, add onion, stir and cook for 5 minutes. Add stock and return the chicken to the pot. Add olives, pepperoncini and roasted potatoes, stir and cook for 3 minutes. Add the rest of the garlic, artichokes, basil and the tomatoes, stir, cook for 3 minutes. Divide between plates and serve.

Enjoy!

Nutrition:

Calories: 221 Cal Fat: 2 g

Fiber: 3 g Carbs: 8 g Protein: 11 g

38. Paprika Chicken Mix

Preparation time: 10 minutes

Cooking time: 30 minutes

Servings: 4

Ingredients: 1/3 cup mustard

Salt and black pepper to the taste

1 cup yellow onion, chopped

1 tablespoon olive oil

1 and ½ cups chicken stock

4 chicken breasts, skinless and boneless

¼ teaspoon sweet paprika

Directions:

In a bowl, whisk the paprika with mustard, salt and pepper. Spread the mix over the chicken and rub well. Heat up a pan with the oil over medium-high heat, add chicken breasts and cook for 2 minutes on each side then transfer to a plate. Heat up the pan once again over medium-high heat, add stock, stir and bring to a simmer. Add onions, salt, pepper and return the chicken to the pan as well. Stir the mix and bring to a simmer over medium heat for 20 minutes, turning meat halfway. Divide between plates, drizzle the sauce over it and serve.

Enjoy!

Nutrition:

Calories: 223 Cal Fat: 8 g

Fiber: 1 g Carbs: 3 gProtein: 15 g

39. Veggie Lunch Salad

Preparation time: 10 minutes

Cooking time: 0 minutes

Servings: 4

Ingredients: 2 carrots, peeled and grated

1 avocado, pitted, peeled and chopped

½ green cabbage head, shredded

10 strawberries, halved

Salt and black pepper to the taste

¼ teaspoon matcha powder

1 teaspoon maple syrup

2 tablespoons white wine vinegar

1 tablespoon Dijon mustard

¼ cup lemon juice   ¾ cup olive oil

Directions:

In a bowl, whisk together the lemon juice with oil, vinegar, matcha tea powder, maple syrup, mustard, salt and pepper. In a salad bowl, mix avocado with cabbage, strawberries and carrots. Add lemon juice, oil, vinegar, matcha powder, maple syrup, mustard, salt and pepper. Toss well and serve for lunch. Enjoy!

Nutrition: Calories: 211 Cal Fat: 4 g Fiber: 0 Carbs: 8 g Protein: 7 g

40. Grilled Eggplant Lunch Salad

Preparation time: 10 minutes

Cooking time: 20 minutes

Servings: 4

Ingredients:

1 tomato, diced

1 eggplant, pricked

A pinch of salt and black pepper

¼ teaspoon ground turmeric

1½ teaspoons red wine vinegar

½ teaspoon chopped oregano

3 tablespoons olive oil

2 garlic cloves, minced

3 tablespoons chopped parsley

2 tablespoons chopped capers

Directions:

Heat up your grill over medium-high heat, add eggplant, cook for 15 minutes, turning from time to time, scoop flesh, roughly chop and put in a bowl. Add salt, pepper to the taste, tomatoes, turmeric, garlic, vinegar, oregano, parsley, oil and capers, toss and serve.

Enjoy!

Nutrition:

Calories: 192 Cal

Fat: 7 g

Fiber: 6 g

Carbs: 12 g

Protein: 7 g

41. Eggplant and Avocado Lunch Mix

Preparation time: 10 minutes

Cooking time: 10 minutes

Servings: 4

Ingredients: 1 eggplant, sliced

1 red onion, sliced

2 teaspoons olive oil

1 avocado, pitted and chopped

1 teaspoon mustard

1 tablespoon red wine vinegar

1 tablespoon chopped oregano

1 teaspoon raw honey

A pinch of salt and black pepper

1 tablespoon chopped parsley

Zest of 1 lemon

Directions:

Brush the onion slices and eggplant slices with the olive oil, place them on the preheated kitchen grill, cook for 5 minutes on each side and let cool down. Cut the veggies into cubes, put in a salad bowl, add avocado and toss. In a bowl, mix vinegar with mustard, oregano, honey, olive oil, salt and pepper, whisk well and add to the salad. Toss together and sprinkle the lemon zest and the parsley on top and serve.

Enjoy!

Nutrition:

Calories: 212 Cal Fat: 7 g Fiber: 7 g

Carbs: 12 g Protein: 7 g

42. Eggplant and Egg Mix

Preparation time: 10 minutes

Cooking time: 30 minutes

Servings: 4

Ingredients: 1 big purple eggplant, cubed

12 eggs, hard-boiled, peeled and cubed

Juice of 1 lemon

A pinch of salt and white pepper

1/3 cup pine nuts   ¼ cup mustard

1 cup chopped sun-dried tomatoes

1 cup halved walnuts   ¼ cup olive oil

Directions:

Spread eggplant cubes on a lined baking sheet. In a bowl, whisk together half of the lemon juice with the oil, salt and pepper. Pour the mix over the eggplant cubes, toss to coat, introduce in the oven at 400 degrees F and bake for 30 minutes. In a food processor, mix the rest of the lemon juice, mustard, salt, pepper, walnuts, tomatoes and pine nuts and pulse well. Put the eggs in a bowl, add eggplant cubes, mustard mix, toss to coat well and serve.   Enjoy!

Nutrition: Calories: 213 Cal Fat: 8 g

Fiber: 3 g Carbs: 12 g Protein: 7 g

43. Stuffed Eggplants

Preparation time: 10 minutes

Cooking time: 50 minutes

Servings: 6

Ingredients: 6 baby eggplants, halved

2 garlic cloves, minced

1 pound ground turkey

1 tablespoon chopped oregano

1 tablespoon lemon juice

¼ teaspoon sweet paprika

¼ teaspoon ground turmeric

A pinch of salt and black pepper

2 tablespoons olive oil

Directions:

Heat up a pan with the oil over medium heat, add the ground turkey, stir and cook for 5-6 minutes. Add the oregano, lemon juice, paprika, turmeric, salt and pepper, stir, and cook for 5-6 minutes more. Take off the heat, cool the mix down and stuff the eggplants with this mix. Arrange the stuffed eggplants on a lined baking sheet, bake in the oven at 400 degrees F for 30 minutes then divide between plates and serve.

Enjoy!

Nutrition: Calories 185 Cal Fat: 10 g

Fiber: 3 g Carbs: 10 g Protein: 16 g

44. Veggie Soup

Preparation time: 10 minutes

Cooking time: 30 minutes

Servings: 4

Ingredients: 1 yellow onion, chopped

2 carrots, chopped 6 mushrooms, chopped

1 red chili pepper, chopped

2 celery sticks, chopped

1 tablespoon coconut oil

A pinch of salt and black pepper

4 garlic cloves, minced

4 ounces kale, chopped

1 cup canned tomatoes, chopped

1 zucchini, chopped 1-quart veggie stock

A handful parsley, chopped for serving

Directions:

Heat up a pot with the oil over medium-high heat, add the celery, carrots, onion, salt and black pepper. Stir and cook for 2 minutes. Add chili pepper, garlic, and mushrooms, stir and cook for 2 minutes. Add tomatoes, stock, kale and zucchinis, stir then bring to a simmer. Cook for 25 minutes, divide into bowls, sprinkle the parsley on top and serve.

Enjoy!

Nutrition: Calories: 180 Cal

Fat: 2 g Fiber: 2 g Carbs: 7 g Protein: 5 g

45. Shrimp Soup

Preparation time: 10 minutes

Cooking time: 30 minutes

Servings: 4

Ingredients:

5 tablespoons curry paste

1 tablespoon coconut oil

1 big chicken breast, cut into thin strips

4 tablespoons coconut aminos

2 cups chicken stock

Juice of 1 lime 1 ½ cups coconut milk

1-pound shrimp, peeled and deveined

½ cup coconut cream

1 broccoli head, florets separated

1 zucchini, chopped 1 carrot, chopped

1 tablespoon parsley, chopped

Directions: Heat up a pot with the oil over medium heat, add curry paste, stir and cook for 1 minute. Add chicken, stock and lime juice. Stir and cook for 2 minutes. Add coconut cream, aminos and coconut milk, stir and cook for 10 minutes. Add broccoli florets, carrots, shrimp and zucchini, stir and cook for 4 minutes. Ladle into bowls, top with parsley and serve. Enjoy!

Nutrition: Calories: 190 Cal

Fat: 3 g Fiber: 2 g Carbs: 6 g Protein: 8 g

46. Chicken and Veggies

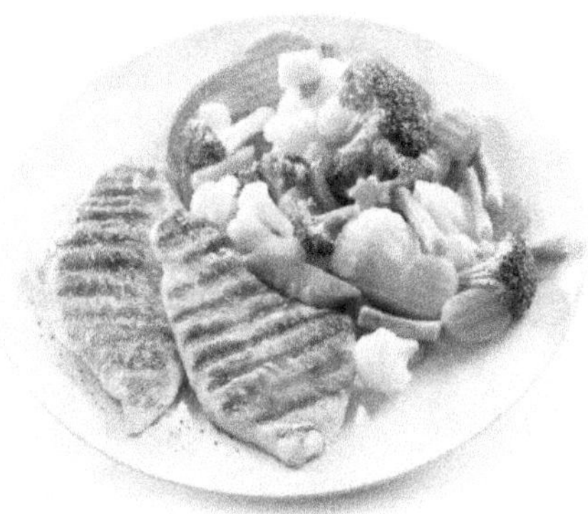

Preparation Time: 10 mins

Cooking Time: 5mins

Servings: 4

Ingredients: ½ c. chopped yellow onion

16 oz. cauliflower florets

2 tbsps. Organic olive oil

½ tsp. Italian seasoning

14 oz. chopped no-salt-added canned tomatoes

4 de-boned, skinless and cubed chicken breasts

¼ tsp. black pepper

Directions:

Heat up a pan while using the oil over medium-high heat, add chicken, black pepper, onion and Italian seasoning, toss and cook for 5 minutes. Add tomatoes and cauliflower, toss, cover the pan and cook over medium heat for twenty possibly even minutes. Toss again, divide everything between plates and serve.

Enjoy!

Nutrition: Calories: 310 Cal

Fat: 6 g Carbs: 14 g Protein: 20 g

Sugars: 6 g Sodium: 550 mg

47. Hidden Valley Chicken Drummies

Preparation Time: 15 mins

Cooking: 30mins

Servings: 6 - 8

Ingredients:

2 tbsps. Hot sauce

½ c. melted butter

Celery sticks

2 packages Hidden Valley dressing dry mix

3 tbsps. Vinegar

12 chicken drumsticks

Paprika

Directions:

Preheat the oven to 350 0F.

Rinse and pat dry the chicken.

In a bowl blend the dry dressing, melted butter, vinegar and hot sauce. Stir until combined.

Place the drumsticks in a large plastic baggie, pour the sauce over drumsticks. Massage the sauce until the drumsticks are coated.

Place the chicken in a single layer on a baking dish. Sprinkle with paprika.

Bake for 30 minutes, flipping halfway.

Serve with crudité or salad.

Nutrition:

Calories: 155 Cal Fat: 18 g

Carbs: 96 g Protein: 15 g Sugars: 0.7 g

Sodium: 340 mg

48. Lemon-Parsley Chicken Breast

Preparation Time: 15 mins

Cooking Time: 11 mins

Servings: 2

Ingredients:

1/3 c. lemon juice

¼ c. fresh parsley

1/3 c. white wine

3 tbsps. Bread crumbs

2 skinless and boneless chicken breasts

2 minced garlic cloves

2 tbsps. Flavorless oil

Directions:

Combine the wine, lemon juice and garlic in a measuring cup.

Pound each chicken breast, until they are ¼ inch thick.

Coat the chicken with bread crumbs, and heat the oil in a large skillet.

Fry the chicken for 6 minutes on each side, until they turn brown.

Stir in the wine mixture over the chicken.

Simmer for 5 minutes

Serve. Pour any extra juices over the chicken. Garnish with parsley.

Nutrition:

Calories: 117 Cal Fat: 12 g

Carbs:7 4 Protein: 14 gSugars: 5.8 g

Sodium: 0

49. Lemony Mussels

Preparation Time: 5 mins

Cooking time: 0

Servings: 4

Ingredients:

1 tbsp. extra virgin extra virgin olive oil

2 minced garlic cloves

2 lbs. scrubbed mussels

Juice of one lemon

Directions:

Put some water in a pot, add mussels, bring with a boil over medium heat, cook for 5 minutes, discard unopened mussels and transfer them with a bowl.

In another bowl, mix the oil with garlic and freshly squeezed lemon juice, whisk well, and add over the mussels, toss and serve.

Enjoy!

Nutrition:

Calories: 140 Cal

Fat: 4 g

Carbs: 8 g

Protein: 8 g

Sugars: 4 g

Sodium: 600 mg

50. Hot Tuna Steak

Preparation Time: 15 mins

Cooking Time: 5 mins

Servings: 6

Ingredients: 2 tbsps. Fresh lemon juice

Pepper. Roasted orange garlic mayonnaise

¼ c. whole black peppercorns

6 sliced tuna steaks

2 tbsps. Extra-virgin olive oil

Salt

Directions:

Place the tuna in a bowl to fit. Add the oil, lemon juice, salt and pepper. Turn the tuna to coat well in the marinade. Let rest 15 to 20 minutes, turning once. Place the peppercorns in a double thickness of plastic bags. Tap the peppercorns with a heavy saucepan or small mallet to crush them coarsely. Place on a large plate. When ready to cook the tuna, dip the edges into the crushed peppercorns. Heat a nonstick skillet over medium heat. Sear the tuna steaks, in batches if necessary, for 4 minutes per side for medium-rare fish, adding 2 to 3 tablespoons of the marinade to the skillet if necessary, to prevent sticking. Serve dolloped with roasted orange garlic mayonnaise

Nutrition: Calories: 124 Cal Fat: 0.4 g

Carbs: 0.6 g Protein: 28 g Sugars: 0 Sodium: 77 mg

51. Marinated Fish Steaks

Preparation Time: 10 mins

Cooking Time: 10 mins

Servings: 4

Ingredients: 4 lime wedges

2 tbsps. Lime juice

2 minced garlic cloves 2 tsps. Olive oil

1 tbsp. snipped fresh oregano

1 lb. fresh swordfish

1 tsp. lemon-pepper seasoning

Directions:

Rinse fish steaks; pat dry wi th paper towels. Cut into four serving size pieces, if necessary.

In a shallow dish combine lime juice, oregano, oil, lemon-pepper seasoning, and garlic. Add fish; turn to coat with marinade. Cover and marinate in refrigerator for 30 minutes to 1-1/2 hours, turning steaks occasionally. Drain fish, reserving marinade. Place fish on the greased unheated rack of a broiler pan. Broil 4 inches from the heat for 8 to 12 minutes or until fish begins to flake when tested with a fork, turning once and brushing with reserved marinade halfway through cooking. Discard any remaining marinade.   Before serving, squeeze the juice from one lime wedge over each steak.

Nutrition: Calories: 240 CalFat: 6 g Carbs: 19 g Protein: 12 g Sugars: 3.27 g Sodium: 325 mg

52. Lime Pork and Green Beans

Preparation time: 10 minutes

Cooking time: 40 minutes

Servings: 4

Ingredients:

2 pounds pork stew meat, cubed

2 tablespoons avocado oil

½ cup green beans, trimmed and halved

2 tablespoons lime juice

1 cup coconut milk

1 tablespoon rosemary, chopped

A pinch of salt and black pepper

Directions:

Heat up a pan with the oil over medium heat, add the meat and brown for 5 minutes.

Add the rest of the ingredients, toss gently, bring to a simmer and cook over medium heat for 35 minutes more.

Divide the mix between plates and serve.

Nutrition:

Calories: 260 Cal

Fat: 5 g

Fiber: 8 g

Carbs: 9 g

Protein: 13 g

53. Pork with Lemongrass

Preparation time: 10 minutes

Cooking time: 30 minutes

Servings: 4

Ingredients:

4 pork chops

2 tablespoons olive oil

2 spring onions, chopped

A pinch of salt and black pepper

½ cup vegetable stock

1 stalk lemongrass, chopped

2 tablespoons coconut aminos

2 tablespoons cilantro, chopped

Directions:

Heat up a pan with the oil over medium-high heat, add the spring onions and the meat and brown for 5 minutes.

Add the rest of the ingredients, toss, and cook everything over medium heat for 25 minutes more.

Divide the mix between plates and serve.

Nutrition:

Calories: 290 Cal

Fat: 4 g

Fiber: 6 g Carbs: 8 g

Protein: 14 g

54. Pork with Olives

Preparation time: 10 minutes

Cooking time: 40 minutes

Servings: 4

Ingredients:

1 yellow onion, chopped

4 pork chops

2 tablespoons olive oil

1 tablespoon sweet paprika

2 tablespoons balsamic vinegar

¼ cup kalamata olives, pitted and chopped

1 tablespoon cilantro, chopped

A pinch of sea salt and black pepper

Directions:

Heat up a pan with the oil over medium heat, add the onion and sauté for 5 minutes.

Add the meat and brown for 5 minutes more.

Add the rest of the ingredients, toss, cook over medium heat for 30 minutes, divide between plates and serve.

Nutrition:

Calories: 280 Cal

Fat: 11 g Fiber: 6 g

Carbs: 10 g Protein: 21 g

55. Pork Chops with Tomato Salsa

Preparation time: 10 minutes

Cooking time: 15 minutes

Servings: 4

Ingredients: 4 pork chops

1 tablespoon olive oil 4 scallions, chopped

1 teaspoon cumin, ground

½ tablespoon hot paprika

1 teaspoon garlic powder

A pinch of sea salt and black pepper

1 small red onion, chopped

2 tomatoes, cubed 2 tablespoons lime juice

1 jalapeno, chopped

¼ cup cilantro, chopped

1 tablespoon lime juice

Directions:

Heat up a pan with the oil over medium heat, add the scallions and sauté for 5 minutes.

Add the meat, cumin paprika, garlic powder, salt and pepper, toss, cook for 5 minutes on each side and divide between plates.

In a bowl, combine the tomatoes with the remaining ingredients, toss, divide next to the pork chops and serve.

Nutrition: Calories: 31 Cal Fat: 23.7 g

Fiber: 1.7 g Carbs: 5.9 g Protein: 19.2 g

56. Cabbage Orange Salad with Citrusy Vinaigrette

Preparation Time: 10 mins

Cooking Time: 0 mins

Servings: 8

Ingredients: 1 teaspoon orange zest,grated

2 tablespoons vegetable stock,reduced-sodium

1 teaspoon each cider vinegar

4 cups red cabbage, shredded

1 teaspoon lemon juice

1 fennel bulb, sliced thinly

1 teaspoon balsamic vinegar

1 teaspoon raspberry vinegar

2 tablespoons of fresh orange juice

2 oranges, peeled, sliced into pieces

1 tablespoon of honey

1/4 teaspoon of salt

Freshly ground pepper

4 teaspoons of olive oil

Directions:

Put the following in a bowl and whisk — lemon juice, orange zest, cider vinegar, salt and pepper, broth, oil, honey, orange juice, balsamic vinegar and raspberry vinegar.

Extract the oranges, fennel and cabbage. Toss to coat.

Nutrition: Calories: 38 Cal

Fat: 3 g Carbohydrates: 12 g Protein: 5 g

57. Lemon Buttery Shrimp Rice

Preparation Time: 10 mins

Cooking Time: 15 mins

Servings: 8

Ingredients:

¼ cup wild rice, cooked according to package instructions

½ tsp. butter, divided

¼ tsp. olive oil

1 cup raw shrimps, shelled, deveined, drained

¼ cup frozen peas, thawed, rinsed, drained

1 Tbsp. lemon juice, freshly squeezed

1 Tbsp. chives, minced

Pinch of sea salt, to taste

Directions:

Pour ¼ tsp. butter and oil into wok set over medium heat. Add in shrimps and peas. Sauté until shrimps are coral pink, about 5 to 7 minutes.

Add in wild rice and cook until well heated through. Season with salt and butter.

Transfer to a plate. Sprinkle chives and lemon juice on top. Serve.

Nutrition: Calories: 80 Cal Fat: 6 g

Carbohydrates: 12 g Protein: 5 g

58. Valencia Salad

Preparation Time: 10 mins

Cooking Time: 0 mins

Servings: 10

Ingredients:

1 tsp. Kalamata olives in oil, pitted, drained lightly, halved, julienned

1 head, small Romaine lettuce, rinsed, spun-dried, sliced into bite-sized pieces

½ piece, small shallot, julienned

1 tsp. Dijon mustard

½ small satsuma or tangerine, pulp only

1 tsp. white wine vinegar

1 tsp. extra virgin olive oil

1 pinch fresh thyme, minced

Pinch of sea salt

Pinch of black pepper, to taste

Directions:

Combine vinegar, oil, fresh thyme, salt, mustard, black pepper, and honey, if using. Whisk well until dressing emulsifies a little.

Toss together remaining salad ingredients in a salad bowl.

Drizzle dressing on top when about to serve. Serve immediately with 1 slice if sugar-free sourdough bread or saltine.

Nutrition: Calories: 30 Cal Fat: 36 g

Carbohydrates: 12 g Protein: 5 g

59. Tenderloin Stir Fry with Red And Green Grapes

Preparation Time: 15 mins

Cooking Time: 25 mins

Servings: 4

Ingredients:

1 medallion, 6 oz. pork tenderloin, trimmed well, remove membrane

sea salt sesame oil

For grape vinaigrette

¼ cup green grapes, quartered

¼ cup red grapes, quartered

black peppercorns, freshly cracked

1 tsp. apple cider vinegar, freshly juiced

Directions:

To make the vinaigrette, toss ingredients in a bowl. Chill prior to serving.

Meanwhile, preheat stovetop or electric grill for at least 3 minutes.

Lightly season pork with salt and sesame oil. Grill only until well seared on both sides, about 10 to 12 minutes. Remove from grill. Tent with aluminium foil, and allow the meat to rest 5 minutes.

Place cooked pork medallion on a plate. Top off with vinaigrette. Serve.

Nutrition: Calories: 133 Cal

Fat:26 g Carbohydrates: 14 g

Protein: 6 g

60. Aioli with Eggs

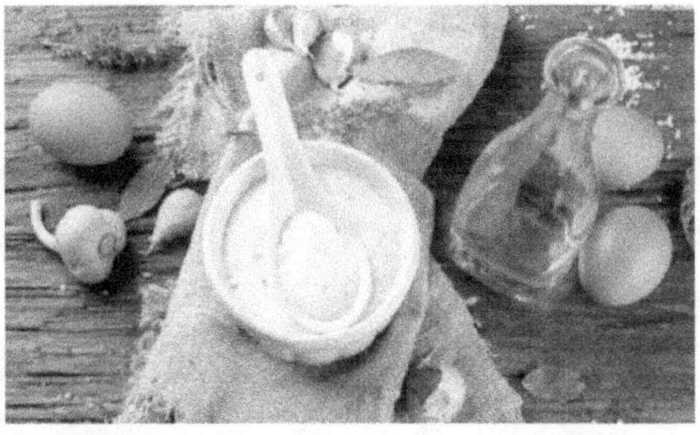

Preparation Time: 20 mins

Cooking Time: 0

Servings: 12

Ingredients:

2 egg yolks

1 garlic, grated

2 Tbsp. water

½ cup extra virgin olive oil

¼ cup lemon juice, fresh squeezed, pips removed

¼ tsp. sea salt

Dash of cayenne pepper powder

Pinch of white pepper, to taste

Directions:

Pour garlic, egg yolks, salt and water into blender; process until smooth. Drizzle in olive oil in a slow stream until dressing emulsifies.

Add in remaining ingredients. Taste; adjust seasoning if needed. Pour into an airtight container; use as needed.

Nutrition: Calories: 220 Cal

Fat: 28 g Carbohydrates: 15 g Protein: 8 g

Snacks Recipes

61. Simple Yet Effective Vegan Truffle

Preparation Time: 20 minutes

Cooking Time: 10 minutes

Servings: 4

1 and a ¼ cups unsweetened coconut, shredded

2 cups of Mejdool dates

1 cup of raw almonds

2 and a ¼ cups of raw cocoa powder

½ a cup of cocoa nibs

½ a cup of agave nectar

2 teaspoons of vanilla extract

1 teaspoon of salt

Directions:

Pre-heat your oven to 350-degree Fahrenheit

Spread out the coconut on a baking sheet

Line another baking sheet with parchment paper

Bake the coconut in your oven for about 7 minutes, making sure to keep stirring them from time to time

Take a food processor and add dates, almonds and process until smooth

Add cocoa powder and process until mixed well

Transfer mix to a bowl

Fold 1 cup of your toasted coconut, agave nectar, salt and vanilla extract into the date mix. Mix well

Roll up the dough into tablespoon sized balls and roll them in the remaining toasted truffle balls.

Transfer the balls to your parchment lined baking sheet and allow them to harden for about 60 minutes

Enjoy!

Nutrition: Calories: 26 Cal

Fats: 0 Carbs: 5 g Protein: 0

62. Guilt and Dairy "Free" Chocolate Pudding

Preparation Time: 10 minutes

Cooking Time: 10 minutes

Servings: 4

Ingredients: 3 tablespoons of cornstarch

2 tablespoons of water

1 and a ½ cups of soy milk

¼ teaspoon of vanilla extract

¼ cup of white sugar

¼ cup of unsweetened cocoa powder

Directions:

Take a small sized bowl and add cornstarch and water and mix well to form a nice paste like texture

Take a large sized saucepan and place it over medium heat

Add soy milk, sugar, vanilla, cocoa and your prepared cornstarch mixture

Give the whole mixture a stir and allow it to cook until boiling point is reached

Keep stirring until the mixture is thick

Remove the heat Allow it to cool and chill in your fridge until it is fully cooled and has settled in Enjoy!

Nutrition: Calories: 267 Cal Fats: 5 g Carbs:53 g Protein:8 g

63. A Very Subtle Cherry Crisp

Preparation Time: 10 minutes

Cooking Time: 30 minutes

Servings: 4

Ingredients: 21 ounce of cherry pie filling

½ a cup of all-purpose flour

½ a cup of rolled oats 2/3 cup of brown sugar

¾ teaspoon cinnamon, ground

¾ teaspoon of nutmeg, ground

¼ cup pecans, chopped

1/3 cup of melted margarine

Directions:

Pre-heat your oven to 350-degree Fahrenheit

Take a 2-quart baking dish and carefully grease it up. Pour the pie filling mixture evenly into the dish and spread it up Take a medium sized bowl and add flour, sugar, oats, cinnamon and nutmeg

Add melted margarine and mix, spread this mixture over your pie filling. Sprinkle chopped up pecans

Bake for 30 minutes until the top shows a golden-brown texture

Allow it to cool for about 15 minutes and enjoy!

Nutrition: Calories: 362 Cal

Fats: 14 g Carbs:57 g Protein:2.9 g

64. Delicious Pumpkin Pie "Spicy" Pastries

Preparation Time: 10 minutes

Cooking Time: 8 minutes

Servings: 25

Ingredients:

½ a pack of rolled up unbaked pie crust (Vegan Compliant)

1 tablespoon of melted Vegan butter

2 tablespoons of packed brown sugar

½ and a 1 teaspoon of pumpkin pie spice

How To

Pre-heat you oven to a temperature of 400 degree Fahrenheit

Unroll the pie crust according to the package direction following the microwave method. Place it on a lightly flour surface

Brush up the pie crust with melted butter

Sprinkle with pie spice and brown sugar

Take a pizza cutter and cut up the dough into ½ inch squares. Take an ungreased large cookie sheet and transfer them to the sheet, making sure to leave some space between the pieces. Bake for about 8 minutes until they are golden brown. Serve and enjoy!

Nutrition: Calories: 46 Cal Fat: 1 g

Carbohydrates: 5 g Protein: 0

65. Cool And Warm Oven Roasted Plums

Preparation Time: 10 minutes

Cooking Time: 15 minutes

Servings: 3

Ingredients: ½ a cup of orange juice

4 pieces of plums, pitted and halved

2 tablespoons of packed brown sugar

½ a teaspoon of cinnamon, ground

1/8 teaspoon of nutmeg, ground

1/8 teaspoon of cumin

1/8 teaspoon of cardamom

¼ cup of toasted and slivered almonds

Cook Directions

Pre-heat your oven to 400-degree Fahrenheit

Take a shallow baking dish and grease it with Cook spray. Add your plums to the pan with the cut side facing up

Take a bowl and whisk in orange juice, cinnamon, brown sugar, cumin, nutmeg and cardamom. Drizzle the mixture over your plums. Bake for 20 minutes until the plums are hot and the sauce shows a bubbly texture

Top with some almonds and enjoy!

Nutrition:

Calories: 113 Cal Fats: 4 g Carbs: 20 g

Protein: 2.1 g

66. Apples With A Fire Within

Preparation Time: 5 minutes

Cooking Time: 10 minutes

Servings: 2

Ingredients:

Cored granny smith apple

1 tablespoon of brown sugar

¼ teaspoon of ground cinnamon

Cook Directions

Core the apples well and fill them up with cinnamon and brown sugar

Wrap the apples using a large piece of heavy foil(making sure to make a few extra twist to make a handle)

Place the apples in a coal of campfire (or BBQ) and allow them to cook for about 5-10 minutes

Gently unwrap the apples and serve!

Nutrition:

Calories: 114 Cal

Fats: 0

Carbs: 30 g

Protein: 0.5 g

67. Awesome and Crunchy Muffins

Preparation Time: 10 minutes

Cooking Time: 30 minutes

Servings: 4

Ingredients:

2 and a ½ cups of coconut milk

1 tablespoon of water

1 and a ¼ cup of white rice flour

2 cups of coconut, unsweetened, shredded

1 teaspoon of salt

1 tablespoon of white sugar

Directions

Pre-heat your oven to 375 degree Fahrenheit

Take mini muffin tins and spray with Cook spray

Take a bowl and add coconut milk and water

Stir in white rice flour, salt and shredded coconut

Spoon up the mixture into your prepped mini muffin cups and sprinkle sugar on top

Bake in your pre-heated oven for 30 minutes until the tops are golden brown

Enjoy!

Nutrition: Calories: 94 Cal

Fats: 8 g Carbs: 7 g

Protein: 1 g

68. The Cherry Beet Delight

Preparation Time: 5 minutes

Cooking Time: 0

Servings: 2

Ingredients 1 cup cherries, pitted

½ cup beets Few banana slices

1 cup water, filtered, alkaline

1 cup coconut milk

Pinch of organic vanilla powder

Pinch of cinnamon

Pinch of stevia

Few mint leaves/lime slices to garnish h

Directions:

Add berries, beets, water, banana slices, coconut milk to your blender

Blend well until smooth

Add more water if the texture is too creamy for you

Add coconut oil, vanilla, cinnamon and stir

Add a bit of stevia for extra sweetness

Garnish with mint leaves and lime slices

Enjoy!

Nutrition: Calories: 200 Cal

Fat: 1 0 g Carbohydrates: 14 g

Protein 2 g

69. Green Delight

Preparation Time: 10 minutes

Cooking Time: 0

Servings: 1

Ingredients:

¾ cup whole almond milk yogurt

2 cups 5 – lettuce mix salad greens

1 pack stevia

1 tablespoon MCT oil

1 tablespoon chia seeds

1 and ½ cups water

Directions:

Add listed Ingredients to blender

Blend until you have a smooth and creamy texture

Serve chilled and enjoy!

Nutrition:

Calories: 320 Cal

Fat: 24 g

Carbohydrates: 17 g

Protein: 10 g

70. Easy Chia Seed Pumpkin Pudding

Preparation Time: 10-15 minutes

Cooking Time: 0

Servings: 4

Ingredients

1 cup pure maple syrup

2 teaspoons pumpkin spice

1 cup pumpkin puree

1 and ¼ cup almond milk

½ cup chia seeds

Directions:

Add all of the ingredients to a bowl and gently stir

Let it refrigerate overnight or for at least 15 minutes

Top with your desired ingredients such as blueberries, almonds, etc.

Serve and enjoy!

Nutrition:

Calories: 230 Cal

Fat: 10 g

Carbohydrates:22 g

Protein:11 g

71. The Mediterranean Fruit Granita

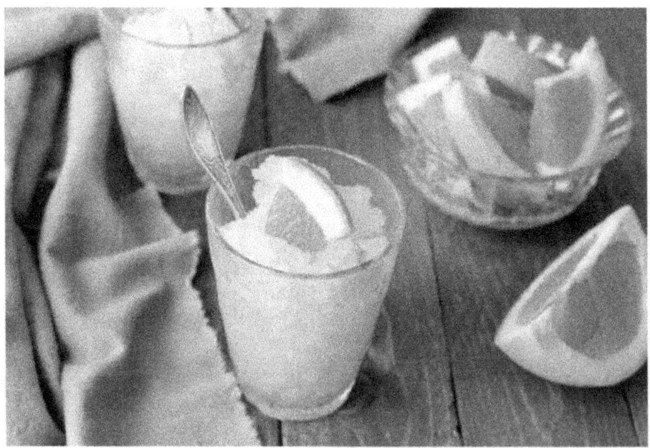

Preparation Time: 5 minutes/30 minutes

Cooking Time: 10-15 minutes

Servings: 4

Ingredients   1-pound ripe nectarines

¼ cup orange juice 2 tablespoons lemon juice

½ cup raspberries   ½ cup brown sugar

Directions

Take a pan and a place it over medium-high heat

Add water and sugar, add the fruits and bring to a boil. Boil everything for 10 minutes. Stir in raspberries. Add juice and extra sugar if needed. Remove the heat and transfer the mixture to your fridge, let it chill for 30 minutes

Serve and enjoy!

Nutrition: Calories: 158 Cal Fat: 40 g

Carbohydrates:0 Protein:14 g

72. Guilt Free Lemon And Rosemary Drink

Preparation Time: 10 minutes

Cooking Time: 0

Servings: 1

Ingredients:

½ cup whole almond milk yogurt

1 cup Garden greens

1 pack stevia

1 tablespoon olive oil

1 stalk fresh rosemary

1 tablespoon lemon juice, fresh

1 tablespoon pepitas

1 tablespoon flaxseed, ground

1 and ½ cups water

Directions:

Add listed Ingredients to blender

Blend until you have a smooth and creamy texture

Serve chilled and enjoy!

Nutrition:

Calories: 312 Cal

Fat: 25 g

Carbohydrates: 14 g

Protein: 9 g

73. Strawberry and Rhubarb Smoothie

Preparation Time: 5 minutes

Cooking Time: 3 minutes

Servings: 1

Ingredients:

1 rhubarb stalk, chopped

1 cup fresh strawberries, sliced

½ cup plain Greek strawberries

Pinch of ground cinnamon

3 ice cubes

Directions:

Take a small saucepan and fill with water over high heat

Bring to boil and add rhubarb, boil for 3 minutes

Drain and transfer to a blender

Add strawberries, honey, yogurt, cinnamon and pulse mixture until smooth

Add ice cubes and blend until thick and has no lumps

Pour into glass and enjoy chilled

Nutrition: Calories: 295 Cal

Fat: 8 g Carbohydrates: 56 g

Protein: 6 g

74. Vanilla Hemp Drink

Preparation Time: 10 minutes

Cooking Time: 0

Servings: 1

Ingredients:

1 cup water

1 cup unsweetened hemp almond milk, vanilla

1 and ½ tablespoons coconut oil, unrefined

½ cup frozen blueberries, mixed

4 cup leafy greens, kale and spinach

1 tablespoons flaxseed

1 tablespoon almond butter

Directions:

Add listed Ingredients to blender

Blend until you have a smooth and creamy texture

Serve chilled and enjoy!

Nutrition:

Calories: 250 Cal

Fat: 20 g

Carbohydrates: 10 g

Protein: 7 g

75. Yogurt and Kale Smoothie

Preparation Time: 10 minutes

Cooking Time: 0

Servings: 1

Ingredients:

1 cup whole almond milk yogurt

1 cup baby kale greens

1 pack stevia

1 tablespoon MCT oil

1 tablespoon sunflower seed

1 cup water

Directions:

Add listed Ingredients to blender

Blend until you have a smooth and creamy texture

Serve chilled and enjoy!

Nutrition:

Calories: 329 Cal

Fat: 26 g

Carbohydrates: 15 g

Protein: 11 g

76. Spiced Kale Chips

Preparation Time: 10 Minutes

Cooking Time: 20 Minutes

Servings: 4

Ingredients:

1 Bunch of Kale, washed & patted dry

1/8 tsp. Garlic Powder

¼ tsp. Salt

1/8 tsp. Black Pepper

¼ tsp. Cayenne Pepper, grounded

1 tsp. Oil

Directions:

Preheat the oven to 300 ° F.

After that, tear off the kale leaves and place them on a wire rack, which is on top of a foil-lined baking sheet.

Now, apply oil in your hands and massage them on the leaves. Tip: You need to use the oil only lightly.

Top it with salt, pepper, and cayenne pepper.

Finally, bake them for 20 minutes or until the edges are crispy.

Tip: If you wish it to be spicier, you can add more cayenne pepper.

Nutrition: Calories: 250 Cal   Proteins:1 g

Carbohydrates: 3 g   Fat: 1 g

77. Vegetable Nuggets

Preparation Time: 10 Minutes

Cooking Time: 25 Minutes

Servings: Makes 24

Ingredients: ¼ tsp. Black Pepper

2 cups Cauliflower Florets

1 Egg, large & pastured

2 cups Broccoli Florets ½ cup Almond Meal

1 cup Carrots, chopped coarsely ¼ tsp. Salt

1 tsp. Garlic, minced

½ tsp. Turmeric, grounded

Directions:

To make these tasty nuggets, you first need to preheat the oven to 400 ° F. Next, place broccoli, turmeric, cauliflower, black pepper, carrots, sea salt, and turmeric in a food processor. Pulse them for a minute or until you get a finely grounded mixture. Then, stir in the almond meal and egg into it and pulse them again until mixed. Now, transfer the veggie-almond mixture to a large mixing bowl. Scoop out the mixture with a tablespoon and make circular discs with your hands. After that, place the discs on the parchment paper-lined baking sheet. Finally, bake them for 20 to 25 minutes while flipping it once. Tip: Serve it along with homemade ranch sauce.

Nutrition: Calories: 220 Cal   Proteins:1.1g
Carbohydrates: 2.1g   Fat: 1.2g

78. Cabbage Pineapple Slaw

Preparation Time: 10 Minutes

Cooking Time: 35 Minutes

Servings: 12 to 14

Ingredients:

2 Red Bell Peppers, sliced thinly

½ of 1 Purple Cabbage, thinly sliced

1 cup Cilantro, sliced thinly

½ of 1 Red Cabbage, sliced thinly

3 cups Pineapple, chopped

For the sauce: 1 cup Cashews, soaked

½ tsp. Red Pepper Flakes

½ cup Water 2-inches Ginger

1 tbsp. + 1 tsp. Lime Juice

Salt & Pepper, to taste

Directions:

To begin with, place all the ingredients needed to make the sauce in a high-speed blender until you get a smooth sauce.

After that, place both the cabbage slices, pineapple, and red peppers in a large mixing bowl. Toss well.

To this, spoon in the cashew sauce and toss them again.

Serve immediately or keep in refrigerator until served.

Tip: You can even add tuna or chicken to this salad for a main dish.

Nutrition: Calories: 220 Cal Proteins:1.1 g

Carbohydrates: 2.1 g   Fat: 1.2 g

79. Turmeric Muffins

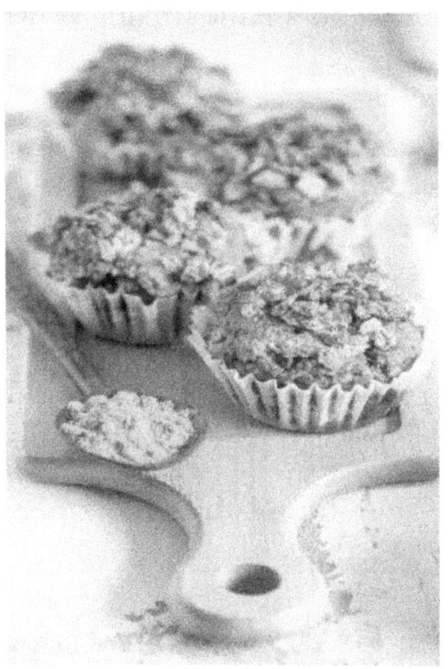

Preparation Time: 10 Minutes

Cooking Time: 25 Minutes

Servings: Makes 8 Muffins

Ingredients:

¾ cup + 2 tbsp. Coconut Flour

6 Eggs, large & preferably pastured

½ tsp. Ginger Powder

½ cup Coconut Milk, unsweetened

Dash of Salt & Pepper

1/3 cup Maple Syrup

½ tsp. Baking Soda

1 tsp. Vanilla Extract

2 tsp. Turmeric

Directions:

Preheat the oven to 350 ° F.

After that, mix eggs, vanilla extract, milk, maple syrup, and milk in a large mixing bowl until combined well.

In another bowl, combine turmeric, coconut flour, ginger powder, baking soda, pepper, and salt.

Now, stir in the coconut flour mixture gradually to the milk mixture until you get a smooth batter.

Then, pour the smooth mixture to paper-lined muffin pan while distributing it evenly.

Finally, bake them for 20 to 25 minutes or until slightly browned at the edges.

Allow the muffins to cool completely.

Tip: They are freezer friendly and stay good for one month.

Nutrition: Calories: 220 Cal

Proteins:1.1 g Carbohydrates: 2.1 g Fat: 1.2 g

80. Coffee Protein Bars

Preparation Time: 10 Minutes

Cooking Time: 10 Minutes

Servings: 12

Ingredients: 2 cups Nuts 5 tbsp. Water

1 cup Egg White Protein Powder

18 Medjool Dates, large & pitted

¼ cup Cocoa Powder, unsweetened

3 tbsp. Instant Coffee

Directions:

First, blend nuts, instant coffee, egg white protein powder, and cocoa in a food processor until broken down into smaller pieces. Tip: Make sure not to over-process them.

After that, stir in the dates and process them again.

Then, spoon in one tablespoon of water gradually to the processor while it is running or until you get a sticky mixture.

Now, transfer the mixture to a parchment paper-lined baking sheet and spread it across evenly. Next, place the baking sheet in the refrigerator for 1 hour or until set. Slice them into bars. Tip: If you prefer, you can add cacao nibs.

Nutrition: Calories: 196 Cal   Proteins:11 g

Carbohydrates: 23 g   Fat: 8 g

81. Cauliflower Popcorn

Preparation Time: 10 Minutes

Cooking Time: 25 Minutes

Servings: 1

Ingredients:

4 cups Cauliflower, broken into florets

Salt, as needed

2 tsp. Extra Virgin Olive Oil

Directions:

First, toss together the cauliflower florets and extra virgin olive oil in a large mixing bowl until coated well.

To this, spoon in the salt and toss well.

Next, bake them for 28 to 30 minutes at 450 ° F or until browned and tender.

Serve with more extra olive oil if needed.

Tip: You can even add cayenne pepper to it if you prefer to make it spicy.

Nutrition:

Calories: 90 Cal

Proteins:4 g

Carbohydrates: 10 g

Fat: 5 g

82. Spiced Pumpkin Seeds

Preparation Time: 10 Minutes

Cooking Time: 15 Minutes

Servings: Makes 1 cup

Ingredients: 1 cup Pumpkin Seeds

1 tsp. Celtic Sea Salt   2 tsp. Olive Oil

1 tbsp. Chili Powder

Directions: To start with, keep the pumpkin seeds in a large-sized iron cast skillet over medium-high heat. Roast them for 3 minutes while stirring it frequently.

After that, take the skillet from the heat and to this, spoon in the chili powder and sea salt. Toss well.

Finally, allow it to cool completely and serve.

Tip: You can reduce or increase the chili powder according to your liking.

Nutrition: Calories: 106 Cal   Proteins:4.4 g

Carbohydrates: 3.6 g   Fat: 9.2 g

83. Curry Roasted Chickpeas

Preparation Time: 10 Minutes

Cooking Time: 40 Minutes

Servings: 4

Ingredients:

1 tbsp. Olive Oil

2 tsp. Curry Powder

15 oz. Garbanzo Beans or Chickpeas, washed & drained

½ tsp. Sea Salt

Directions:

First, preheat the oven to 400 ° F.

Next, place the chickpeas, salt, olive oil, and curry powder in a large mixing bowl and combine them well.

Now, transfer the seasoned chickpeas to a baking sheet and spread them in a single layer.

After that, bake them for 25 to 30 minutes or until crispy while turning them once in between.

Allow them to cool completely and serve.

Tip: You can reduce or increase the curry powder according to your spice level.

Nutrition:

Calories: 420 Cal   Proteins:20.7 g

Carbohydrates: 65.1 g   Fat: 10.1 g

84. Coconut Oats Balls

Preparation Time: 10 Minutes

Cooking Time: 40 Minutes

Servings: Makes 50

Ingredients: 2/3 cup Honey

2 cups Steel Oats   2 tsp. Vanilla Extract

1 ½ cup Coconut Flakes, unsweetened

1 cup Almonds, chopped

1 cup Peanut Butter

Directions:

For making these energy balls, you first need to place the oats in the food processor and then process them until broken down.

Next, combine the rest of the ingredients in a large mixing bowl until everything comes together.

Now, by using your hands, make balls out of this smooth dough. Then, place the balls in the refrigerator for half an hour or until set.

Serve and enjoy.

Tip: You can reduce or increase the curry powder according to your spice level.

Nutrition:

Calories: 88 Cal   Proteins:2 g

Carbohydrates: 9 g

Fat: 5 g

85. Seasoned Coconut Flakes

Preparation Time: 5 Minutes

Cooking Time: 5 Minutes

Servings: 2

Ingredients: ¼ tsp. Nutmeg

1 cup Coconut Flakes, unsweetened

1 tsp. Coconut Oil ¼ tsp. Allspice

1 tsp. Cinnamon ¼ tsp. Salt

Directions:

Preheat the oven to 350 ° F.

After that, place all the ingredients needed to make the savory snacks, excluding the coconut oil in a large zip lock bags. Shake well. Next, spoon in the coconut oil to the bag and shake again, so the seasoning coats the coconut flakes.

Now, transfer the seasoned coconut to a greased baking sheet.

Then, place the sheet in the middle rack and bake the coconut flakes for 4 to 5 minutes. Tip: Make sure not to over bake them.

Finally, remove the sheet from the oven immediately and allow it to cool completely before serving.

Tip: You can add a low-carb sweetener of your choice to it if desired.

Nutrition: Calories: 90 Cal   Proteins:1 g

Carbohydrates: 4.6 g   Fat: 7.8 g

86. Turmeric Bars

Preparation time: 2 hours and 5 minutes

Cooking Time: 10 minutes

Servings 6

Ingredients: 1 cup shredded coconut

10 dates, pitted 1 tablespoon coconut oil

1 teaspoon cinnamon 1 ¼ cup coconut butter

1 ½ teaspoon turmeric powder

2 teaspoons honey

1/8 teaspoon black pepper

Directions:

Prepare a baking pan a nd line with parchment paper.

Place the cocon ut and dates in a food processor and pulse unti l well-combined. Add in the coconut oil and cinnamon.

Press the dough at the bottom of the pan and allow to set in the fridge for 2 hours.

Make the filling by melting the coconut butter in a double boiler. Stir in turmeric powder and honey. Pour in the mixtu reinto the pan with the crust.

Allow to set in the fridge for at least 2 hours.

Nutrition:

Calories 410 Cal Fat 41 g Carbs 13 g

Protein 1 g Fiber: 2 g

87. Anti-Inflammatory Turmeric Gummies

Preparation time: 4 hours

Cooking Time: 10 minutes

Servings 6

Ingredients:

1 teaspoon ground turmeric

6 tablespoons maple syrup

8 tablespoons unflavored gelatin powder

3 ½ cups water

Directions:

In a pot, combine the water, turmeric, and maple syrup.

Bring to a boil for 5 minutes.

Remove from the heat and sprinkle with gelatin powder. Mix to hydrate the gelatin.

Turn on the heat and bring to a boil until the gelatin is completely dissolved.

Pour the mixture in a dish and chill the mixture in the fridge for at least 4 hours.

Once set, slice into small squares.

Nutrition:

Calories 68 Cal

Fat 0.03 g

Carbs 17 g

Protein 0.2 g Fiber: 0.1 g

88. Ginger Spiced Mixed Nuts

Preparation time: 5 minutes

Cooking Time: 40 minutes

Servings: 4

Ingredients:

2 large egg whites, pasture-raised

2 cups mixed nuts (raw almond, pumpkin seeds, cashew, etc.)

1 teaspoon grated ginger

½ teaspoon salt

Directions:

Preheat the oven to 2500F.

Whip the egg whites until frothy. Add in ginger and salt.

Add in the mixed nuts into the egg mixture. Stir to coat everything.

Place parchment paper in a baking tray and spread the nuts evenly on to the sheet.

Bake for 40 minutes.

Allow the mixture to cool and harden.

Break into pieces and store in the fridge until ready to consume

Nutrition:

Calories 423 Cal

Fat 36 g

Carbs 16 g Protein 17 g Fiber: 9 g

89. Spicy Tuna Rolls

Preparation time: 10 minutes

Cooking Time: 0

Servings: 6

Ingredients: 1 medium cucumber

1 can yellowfin tuna, wild-caught

2 slices avocado, diced

1/8 teaspoon salt 1/8 teaspoon pepper

Directions:

Use a mandolin to thinly slice the cucumber lengthwise.

In a mixing bowl, combine the tuna and avocado. Season with salt and pepper to taste.

Spoon the tuna and avocado mixture and spread evenly on cucumber slices.

Roll the cucumber slices and secure the ends with toothpicks.

Allow to chill in the fridge before serving.

Nutrition:

Calories 135 Cal

Fat 10 g

Carbs 6 g

Protein 7 g

Fiber: 5 g

90. Veggie Burrito

Preparation time: 10 minutes

Cooking Time: 5 minutes

Servings: 2

Ingredients: 1 teaspoon avocado oil

4 medium collard greens, stalks trimmed

1/3 cup bell pepper, julienned

1/3 cup chopped tomatoes

1/3 cup red onions, sliced thinly

¼ cup avocado meat

1 cup cooked quinoa ¼ teaspoon salt

¼ cup cilantro leaves, chopped

Directions:

Bring water to a boil and blanch the collard greens. Set aside. In a skillet, heat the avocado oil over medium flame and sauté the bell pepper for 1 minute. Set aside. Assemble the burrito by placing the blanched collard greens on a flat surface.

Place the bell pepper, tomatoes, onions, avocado meat, and quinoa in the center. Add in the cilantro leaves.

Roll the collard greens to create a burrito.

Nutrition:

Calories 175 Cal Carbs 25 g

Protein 5 g Fiber: 5 g

Dinner Recipes

91. Tasty Turkey Baked Balls

Preparation Time: 10-minutes

Cooking Time: 30-minutes

Servings: 6

Ingredients: 1-pound ground turkey

½-cup fresh breadcrumbs, white or whole wheat

½-cup Parmesan cheese, freshly grated

½-Tbsp basil, freshly chopped

½-Tbsp oregano, freshly chopped

1-pc large egg, beaten

1-Tbsp parsley, freshly chopped

3-Tbsps milk or water

A dash of salt and pepper

A pinch of freshly grated nutmeg

Directions:

Preheat your oven to 350°F. Line two baking pans with parchment paper. Stir in all of the ingredients in a large mixing bowl. Form 1-inch balls from the mixture and place each ball in the baking pan. Put the pan in the oven. Bake for 30 minutes, or until the turkey cooks through and the surfaces turn brown.

Turn the meatballs once halfway into the cooking.

Nutrition: Calories: 517 Cal

Fat: 17.2 g Protein: 38.7 g Carbs: 52.7 g

Fiber: 1 g

92. Chicken, Corn & Spinach Sauté

Preparation Time: 5-minutes

Cooking Time: 20-minutes

Servings: 4

Ingredients: 1-Tbsp olive oil

1-clove garlic, minced

2-pc chicken breasts, sliced ½-cup corn kernels

1-pc zucchini, cubed 1-tsp cumin

2-cups baby spinach leaves

Juice of one lime ¼-cup goat cheese, crumbled

Salt and pepper, to taste

Directions:

Sauté the chicken with garlic and olive oil in a skillet placed over medium high heat Cook for about a minute until the chicken turns brown. Remove the chicken from the pan. Set aside. In the same skillet, add in the corn and zucchini, and cook for a minute until the zucchini is tender. Add the cumin, and stir while cooking further for one more minute. Put the browned chicken back into the skillet, and cook until done. Stir in the lime juice and spinach, and keep cooking until the spinach wilts. Sprinkle with salt and pepper.

Just before serving, stir in the goat cheese.

Nutrition: Calories: 303 Cal

Fat: 10.1 g Protein: 22.7 g Carbs: 32.3 g

Fiber: 2 g

93. Sprouts & Slices In Wheat Wrap

Preparation Time: 10-minutes

Cooking Time: 0

Servings: 2

Ingredients: ¼-cup carrots, grated

½-cup romaine lettuce, shredded

½-pc cucumber, sliced round, then halved

½-cup bean sprouts ¼-cup tomatoes, diced

⅛-cup red onions, diced

¼-cup mozzarella, partly skimmed, shredded

¼-cup hummus or guacamole dressing

1-pc whole-wheat wrap, large

Directions:

In a medium-sized mixing bowl, prepare the dressing or spread by combining all of the ingredients excluding the cheese and wrap. Mix well until thoroughly combined.

On a clean table, spread out the whole-wheat wrap. Spread the dressing evenly on the wrap. Be sure to leave a couple of inches on one end of the wrap for folding.

Add the cheese to an even layer over the spread. Fold over the full wrap and tuck in at the bottom.

Nutrition:

Calories: 226 Cal

Fat: 7.5 g

Protein: 16.9 g

Carbs: 27.6 g

Fiber: 5 g

94. Feta-Filled & Tomato-Topped Turkey Burger Bites

Preparation Time: 10-minutes

Cooking Time: 20-minutes

Servings: 1

Ingredients:

1-lb turkey, lean, ground

½-tsp black pepper

Kosher or sea salt to taste

½-cup tomatoes, sun-dried, diced

½-cup Feta cheese, low fat

2-Tbsps green onions or chives, diced

Directions:

Stir in all the listed ingredients in a mixing bowl. Mix well until blended thoroughly.

Divide the mixture evenly into four patties. Store them in the refrigerator.

When cooking time comes, you can either grill or fry the frozen patties for about 10 minutes each on both sides.

Serve by topping the burgers with your preferred condiments.

Nutrition: Calories: 238 Cal

Fat: 7.9 g Protein: 17.8 g

Carbs: 26.8 g

Fiber: 3g

95. Simply Sautéed Flaky Fillet

Preparation Time: 2-minutes

Cooking Time: 8-minutes

Servings: 6

Ingredients:

6-fillets tilapia

2-Tbsps olive oil

1-pc lemon, juice

Salt and pepper to taste

¼-cup parsley or cilantro, chopped

Directions:

Sauté tilapia fillets with olive oil in a medium-sized skillet placed over medium heat. Cook for 4 minutes on each side until the fish flakes easily with a fork.

Add salt and pepper to taste. Pour the lemon juice to each fillet.

To serve, sprinkle the cooked fillets with chopped parsley or cilantro.

Nutrition:

Calories: 249 Cal

Fat: 8.3 g

Protein: 18.6 g

Carbs: 25.9 g

Fiber: 1 g

96. Spicy Sautéed Chinese Chicken

Preparation Time: 25-minutes

Cooking Time: 5-minutes

Servings: 4

Ingredients: For the Marinade:

1-Tbsp ginger, peeled and minced

1-Tbsp garlic-chili sauce or chili paste

1-Tbsp Hoisin sauce 1-Tbsp light soy sauce

For the Chicken:

1-lb chicken breasts, boneless, skinless, cubed

1½-Tbsps canola oil

Directions:

Whisk all the marinade ingredients altogether in a mixing bowl. Add in the chicken pieces, and toss lightly to coat the chicken uniformly with the marinade. Cover the bowl. Chill in the refrigerator for 20 minutes.

Sauté the chicken pieces with canola oil in a medium-sized pan placed over medium high heat. Cook for about 5 minutes until its juices run clear and cook through. (Cook further if the chicken pieces are large).

To serve, place the cooked chicken over a choice of either cooked quinoa or brown rice noodles, or brown rice.

Nutrition: Calories: 190 Cal

Fat: 6.3 g Protein: 14.2 g Carbs: 21 g

Fiber: 2 g

97. Tasty Thai Chicken in Crisp Cups

Preparation Time: 5-minutes

Cooking Time: 5-minutes

Servings: 6

Ingredients: 1½-Tbsps cooking oil

½-lb chicken breast, ground- - 2-pcs shallots, diced ¼-pc red onion, diced - -1-clove garlic, finely minced

Jalapeño or Fresno chilies, freshly minced

1-Tbsp fish sauce ½-pc lime, juiced

1-tsp soy sauce, reduced-sodium

1-head iceberg lettuce, separated into cups

A handful of cilantro and mint, finely chopped

Directions: Sauté the ground chicken with a tablespoon of olive oil in a large wok placed over high heat. Cook for about 3 minutes until the surfaces of the ground chicken turn brown. Push the browned ground chicken to one side of the wok, and pour in the remaining oil. Add in the shallots, red onion, garlic, and fresh chilies. Sauté these added ingredients for about half a minute until effusing their fragrance. Pour in the sauce, juice of one lime, and soy sauce. Stir the entire mixture, including the ground chicken until cooked thoroughly. To serve, distribute the cooked mixture evenly in lettuce cups.

Nutrition: Calories: 120 Cal Fat: 4 gProtein: 9 g Carbs: 23.8 g Fiber: 1.8 g

98. Zesty Zucchini & Chicken In Classic Santa Fe Stir-Fry

Preparation Time: 5-minutes

Cooking Time: 15-minutes

Servings: 2

Ingredients: 1-Tbsp olive oil

2-pcs chicken breasts, sliced

1-pc onion, small, diced

2-cloves garlic, minced 1-pc zucchini, diced

½- cup carrots, shredded

1-tsp paprika, smoked 1-tsp cumin, ground

½-tsp chili powder ¼-tsp sea salt

2-Tbsp fresh lime juice

¼-cup cilantro, freshly chopped

Brown rice or quinoa, when serving

Directions:

Sauté the chicken with olive oil for about 3 minutes until the chicken turns brown. Set aside. Use the same wok and add the onion and garlic. Cook until the onion is tender. Add in the carrots and zucchini. Stir the mixture, and cook further for about a minute. Add all the seasonings into the mix, and stir to cook for another minute. Return the chicken in the wok, and pour in the lime juice. Stir to cook until everything cooks through.

To serve, place the mixture over cooked rice or quinoa and top with the freshly chopped cilantro.

Nutrition: Calories: 191 CalFat: 5.3 g

Protein: 11.9 g Carbs: 26,3 g Fiber: 2.5 g

99. Crispy Cheese-Crusted Fish Fillet

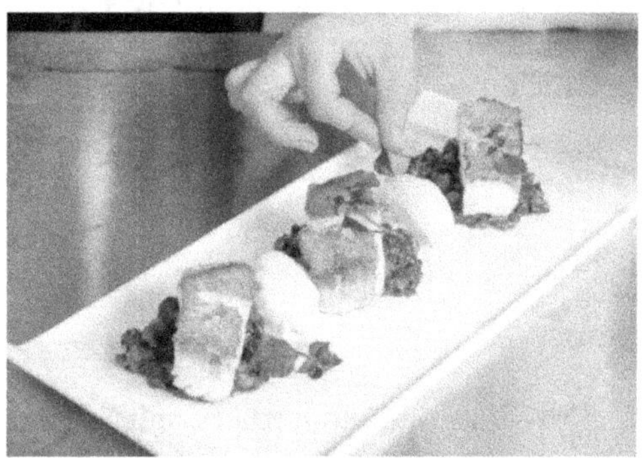

Preparation Time: 5-minutes

Cooking Time: 10-minutes

Servings: 4

Ingredients:

¼-cup whole-wheat breadcrumbs

¼-cup Parmesan cheese, grated

¼-tsp sea salt ¼-tsp ground pepper

1-Tbsp olive oil 4-pcs tilapia fillets

Directions:

Preheat the oven to 375°F.

Stir in the breadcrumbs, Parmesan cheese, salt, pepper, and olive oil in a mixing bowl. Mix well until blended thoroughly.

Coat the fillets with the mixture, and lay each on a lightly sprayed baking sheet. Place the sheet in the oven. Bake for 10 minutes until the fillets cook through and turn brownish.

Nutrition: Calories: 255 Cal

Fat: 7 g Protein: 15.9 g

Carbs: 34. G Fiber: 2.6 g

100. Ambrosial Avocado & Salmon Salad in Lemon-Dressed Layers

Preparation Time: 10-minutes

Cooking Time: 0

Servings: 4

Ingredients:

For the Avocado & Salmon Salad:

6-oz wild salmon 4-units jars

1-pc avocado, pitted, peeled, and diced

2-cups loosely packed salad greens

½-cup Monterey Jack cheese, reduced-fat, shredded

¾-cup tomato, chopped

1-Tbsp lemon juice, freshly squeezed

For the Lemon Dressing:

1 Tbsp lemon juice, freshly squeezed

1 Tbsp olive oil, extra-virgin

1 tsp honey ⅛-tsp Kosher or sea salt

⅛-tsp black pepper ½-tsp Dijon mustard

Directions: Combine and whisk all the dressing ingredients excluding the olive oil in a small mixing bowl. Mix well. Drizzle gradually with the oil into the dressing mixture, and keep whisking while pouring. Pour the dressing as to distribute evenly into each jar. Distribute uniformly into each jar similar amounts of the following ingredients in this order: diced tomatoes, cheese, avocado, salmon, and lettuce. Secure each jar by with its lid, and chill the jars in the fridge until ready for serving.

Nutrition: Calories: 267 Cal Fat: 7.4 g

Protein: 16.6 g Carbs: 38.1 g Fiber: 4.8 g

101. Sautéed Shrimp Jambalaya Jumble

Preparation Time: 15-minutes

Cooking Time: 30-minutes

Servings: 4

Ingredients: 10-oz. medium shrimp, peeled

¼-cup celery, chopped   ½-cup onion, chopped

1-Tbsp oil or butter ¼-tsp garlic, minced

¼-tsp onion salt or sea salt

⅓-cup tomato sauce ½-tsp smoked paprika

½-tsp Worcestershire sauce

⅔-cup carrots, chopped

1¼-cups chicken sausage, precooked and diced

2-cups lentils, soaked overnight and precooked

2-cups okra, chopped

A dash of crushed red pepper and black pepper

Parmesan cheese, grated for topping (optional)

Directions:

Sauté the shrimp, celery, and onion with oil in a pan placed over medium high heat for five minutes, or until the shrimp turn pinkish.

Add in the rest of the ingredients, and sauté further for 10 minutes, or until the veggies are tender.

To serve, divide the jambalaya mixture equally among four serving bowls. Top with pepper and cheese, if desired.

Nutrition: Calories: 529 Cal

Fat: 17.6 g Protein: 26.4 g Carbs: 98.4 g

Fiber: 32.3 g

102. Toasted Tilapia Topped with Panko & Pecans

Preparation Time: 15-minutes

Cooking Time: 18-minutes

Servings: 4

Ingredients: ⅛-tsp salt

⅓-cup pecans, chopped

⅓-cup whole-wheat panko breadcrumbs

½-tsp coconut palm sugar 1½-tsps olive oil

2-tsps chopped fresh rosemary

A pinch of cayenne pepper

1-unit egg white 4 x 4-oz. tilapia fillets

Directions:

Preheat your oven to 350°F. Stir in the first seven ingredients in a small baking dish. Mix well until thoroughly combined.

Put the dish in the oven. Bake for 8 minutes or until the mixture turns brown. Set aside. Increase the heat to 400°F. Meanwhile, grease a large baking dish with cooking spray. Whisk the egg white in a shallow bowl. Dip the fillet, one at a time, in the bowl of whisked egg. Dredge the soaked fillet in the pecan mixture, coating each side lightly. Place each coated fillet in the large baking dish.

Put the dish in the oven, and bake for 10 minutes, or until the fillets cook through.

Nutrition: Calories: 222 Fat: 6.1g Protein: 13.8g Carbs: 29.5g Fiber: 1.8g

103. Tortilla Tostadas with Peppered Potato & Kingly Kale

Preparation Time: 12-minutes

Cooking Time: 10-minutes

Servings: 4

Ingredients:

2-pcs medium sweet potatoes, cleaned and chopped

A pinch of cayenne pepper

3-Tbsps olive oil (divided)

8-stems kale, roughly chopped

A pinch of salt

12-pcs Brussels sprouts, finely chopped

1-tsp honey

1-Tbsp lime juice

Corn tortillas

A drizzle of yogurt

Mint, freshly chopped (optional)

Dried coconut (optional)

Directions:

Preheat your oven to 400°F. Line two baking sheets with aluminum foil.

Toss the sweet potatoes with cayenne pepper and 2-tablespoons of oil on the first baking sheet.

In the other baking sheet, toss the kale with salt and oil.

Put both sheets in the oven. Roast the potatoes for 40 minutes. Roast the kale for 10 minutes until, or until the edges turn crispy, but not browned.

Meanwhile, toss the sprouts with the honey and lime juice. Set aside.

Place the corn tortillas on a piece of tin foil, and toast in the warm oven for 3 minutes.

To serve, scoop equally the sweet potatoes and crispy kale among four tortillas. Top each tortilla with the sprout's slaw. Drizzle with yogurt, mint, and toasted coconut, if desired.

Nutrition:

Calories: 200 Cal Fat: 6.6 g

Protein: 15 g Total Carbs: 24.5 g Fiber: 4.5 g

104. Turkey Tomato Sweet Potato Stuffed Peppers

Preparation Time: 10-minutes

Cooking Time: 50-minutes

Servings: 4

Ingredients:

1-tbsp extra-virgin olive oil

2-cups ground turkey, grass-fed

2-cloves garlic, minced

½-cup onions, diced

1⅔-cups sweet potato, diced

½-cup homemade tomato sauce

Crushed red pepper flakes (optional)

A dash of salt and pepper

2-pcs big bell peppers, sliced in half

Directions:

Preheat your oven to 350°F. Meanwhile, grease a baking dish with cooking spray.

Heat the oil in a skillet placed over medium high heat. Sauté the garlic and turkey for 10 minutes or until the meat is no longer pink, stirring occasionally. (Ensure breaking the ground turkey with a wooden spoon while it cooks.)

Add the onions, and cook further for 3 minutes, or until the onions turn golden brown.

Add the sweet potato, and cover the skillet. Cook the potatoes for 8 minutes, or until they are tender. (Pour more oil or water, as necessary)

Pour the tomato sauce, pepper flakes, and a dash of salt and pepper to taste. Set aside.

Arrange the halved bell peppers in the baking dish, with their cavity sides facing up. Stuff each half with the cooked mixture.

Put the dish in the oven. Roast for half an hour until the bell peppers become tender.

Nutrition:

Calories: 324 Cal

Fat: 10.8 g

Protein: 24.3 g

Carbs: 37 g

Fiber: 4.6 g

105. Baked Buffalo Cauliflower Chunks

Preparation Time: 10-minutes

Cooking Time: 35-minutes

Servings: 2

Ingredients:

¼-cup water

¼-cup banana flour

A pinch of salt and pepper

1-pc medium cauliflower, cut into bite-size pieces

½-cup hot sauce

2-Tbsps butter, melted

Blue cheese or ranch dressing (optional)

Directions:

Preheat your oven to 425°F. Meanwhile, line a baking pan with foil.

Combine the water, flour, and a pinch of salt and pepper in a large mixing bowl. Mix well until thoroughly combined.

Add the cauliflower; toss to coat thoroughly. Transfer the mixture to the baking pan. Bake for 15 minutes, flipping once.

While baking, combine the hot sauce and butter in a small bowl. Pour the sauce over the baked cauliflower.

Return the baked cauliflower to the oven, and bake further for 20 minutes. Serve immediately with a ranch dressing on the side, if desired.

Nutrition: Calories: 168 Cal Fat: 5.6 g

Protein: 8.4 g Carbs: 23.8 g Fiber: 2.8 g

106.   Cool Garbanzo and Spinach Beans

Preparation Time: 5-10 minutes

Cooking Time: 0

Servings: 4

Ingredients

1 tablespoon olive oil

½ onion, diced

10 ounces spinach, chopped

12 ounces garbanzo beans

½ teaspoon cumin

How To

Take a skillet and add olive oil, let it warm over medium-low heat

Add onions, garbanzo and cook for 5 minutes

Stir in spinach, cumin, garbanzo beans and season with salt

Use a spoon to smash gently

Cook thoroughly until heated, enjoy!

Nutrition: Calories: 90 Cal

Fat: 4 g Carbohydrates:11 g Protein:4 g

107.   Lemony Garlic Shrimp

Preparation Time: 5-10 minutes

Cooking Time: 10-15 minutes

Servings: 4

Ingredients

1 and ¼ pounds shrimp, boiled or steamed

3 tablespoons garlic, minced

¼ cup lemon juice

2 tablespoons olive oil

¼ cup parsley

Directions:

Take a small skillet and place it over medium heat, add garlic and oil and stir cook for 1 minute

Add parsley, lemon juice and season with salt and pepper accordingly

Add shrimp in a large bowl and transfer the mixture from the skillet over the shrimp

Chill and serve

Enjoy!

Nutrition:

Calories: 130 Cal

Fat: 3 g

Carbohydrates: 2 g

Protein: 22 g

108. Coconut and Hazelnut Chilled Glass

Preparation Time: 10 minutes

Cooking Time: 0

Servings: 1

Ingredients:

½ cup coconut almond milk

¼ cup hazelnuts, chopped

1 and ½ cups water

1 pack stevia

Directions

Add listed Ingredients to blender

Blend until you have a smooth and creamy texture

Serve chilled and enjoy!

Nutrition:

Calories: 457 Cal

Fat: 46 g

Carbohydrates: 12 g

Protein: 7 g

109. Coriander Greens with Zucchini Sauté!

Preparation Time: 10 minutes

Cooking Time: 10 minutes

Servings: 4

Ingredients

10 ounces beef, sliced into 1-2-inch strips

1 zucchini, cut into 2-inch strips

¼ cup parsley, chopped

3 garlic cloves, minced

2 tablespoons tamari sauce

4 tablespoons avocado oil

Directions:

Add 2 tablespoons avocado oil in a frying pan over high heat

Place strips of beef and brown for a few minutes on high heat

Once the meat is brown, add zucchini strips and Saute until tender

Once tender, add tamari sauce, garlic, parsley and let them sit for a few minutes more

Serve immediately and enjoy!

Nutrition:

Calories: 500 Cal

Fat: 40 g

Carbohydrates: 5 g

Protein: 31 g

110.   Walnuts and Asparagus Delight

Preparation Time: 5 minutes

Cooking Time: 5 minutes

Servings: 4

Ingredients

1 and ½ tablespoons olive oil

¾ pound asparagus, trimmed

¼ cup walnuts, chopped

Sunflower seeds and pepper to taste

Directions

Place a skillet over medium heat add olive oil and let it heat up

Add asparagus, Sauté for 5 minutes until browned

Season with sunflower seeds and pepper

Remove heat

Add walnuts and toss

Serve warm!

Nutrition:

Calories: 124 Cal

Fat: 12 g

Carbohydrates: 2 g

Protein: 3 g

111.   Butternut Squash with Lentils

Preparation time: 15 minutes

Cooking time: 20 minutes

Servings: 6

Ingredients   Coconut oil – 1 Tbsp.

Onion – 1, chopped   Garlic – 2 cloves, minced

Small butternut squash – 1, cut into ½ inch cubes

Packed spinach – 4 cups Salt – 1 tsp.

Ground black pepper – ½ tsp.

Coconut milk – 1 (13.5 ounce) can

Vegetable broth – 1 ½ to 2 cups

Lentils – 1 (15-ounce) can lentils, drained and rinsed

Chopped fresh parsley – ¼ cup

Chopped fresh sage – 2 Tbsps.

Chopped toasted walnuts - ½ cup

Directions:

Preheat the oven to 375F.

Melt the coconut oil in a skillet. Add the garlic and onion. Sauté for 3 minutes.

Add the spinach, butternut squash, salt, and pepper. Sauté for 3 minutes more.

Stir in the coconut milk and just enough vegetable broth to cover the squash. Bring the liquid to a boil.

Add the sage, parsley, and lentils. Stir to combine.

Place the skillet in the preheated oven and bake the casserole for 15 to 20 minutes, until the squash is tender.

Transfer the casserole to a serving dish and garnish with the walnuts.

Nutrition:

Calories: 502 Cal

Fat: 37 g

Carb: 47 g

Protein: 20 g

112.   Buckwheat Noodle Pad Thai

Preparation time: 15 minutes

Cooking time: 15 minutes

Servings: 4

Ingredients

Buckwheat soba noodles – 1 (8-ounce) package

Coconut oil – 1 Tbsp.

Red onion – 1, chopped

Garlic – 2 cloves, minced

Minced fresh ginger – 2 tsps.

Zucchini – 1, chopped

Bok choy – 2, sliced thin

Coconut aminos – 1 Tbsp.

Apple cider vinegar – 1 Tbsp.

Almond butter - 3 Tbsps.

Toasted sesame oil – 2 Tbsps.

Raw honey – 1 Tbsp.

Vegetable broth – ¼ cup

Salt

Scallions – 2, sliced thin

Chopped fresh cilantro – ¼ cup

Sesame seeds – 2 Tbsps.

Directions:

Cook the soba noodles according to the package directions, drain, and set aside.

Melt the coconut oil in a large pan.

Add the garlic, red onion, ginger, zucchini, and bok choy. Sauté for 5 minutes.

Add the cider vinegar, coconut aminos, almond butter, sesame oil, honey, and broth. Cook for 2 minutes. Stirring constantly.

Add the soba noodles and sauté them. Mix with the vegetables.

Season with salt and transfer the Pad Thai to a serving dish.

Garnish with scallions, cilantro, and sesame seeds.

Nutrition:

Calories: 486 Cal

Fat: 21 g

Carb: 63 g

Protein: 19 g

113.   White Beans and Olive Stuffed Zucchinis

Preparation time: 15 minutes

Cooking time: 20 minutes

Servings: 4

Ingredients

Large zucchinis – 4, halved lengthwise, seeds removed

Extra-virgin olive oil – 2 Tbsps. plus additional for brushing

Salt – ½ tsp, plus additional for seasoning

Ground black pepper

Pinch ground rosemary

White beans – 1 (15-ounce) can, drained, and rinsed

Chopped pitted green olives – ½ cup

Garlic – 2 cloves, minced

Chopped arugula – 1 cup

Chopped fresh parsley – ¼ cup

Apple cider vinegar - 1 Tbsp.

Directions:

Preheat the oven to 375F.

Brush a rimmed baking sheet with oil.

Brush the scooped-out section of each zucchini boat with olive oil and lightly season the inside of each boat with salt, pepper, and rosemary.

Transfer the zucchini to the prepared baking sheet, cut-side up.

Place the sheet in the preheated oven and roast for 15 to 20 minutes, or until the zucchini are tender and lightly browned.

In a bowl, lightly mash the white beans with a fork.

Add the garlic, olives, arugula, parsley, cider vinegar, the remaining ½ tsp. salt, and remaining 2 tbsps. olive oil. Season with pepper and mix well.

Spoon the bean mixture into the zucchini boats and serve.

Nutrition: Calories: 269 Cal Fat: 12 g

Carb: 38 g Protein: 13 g

114.   Buckwheat and Sweet Potatoes

Preparation time: 15 minutes

Cook time: 20 minutes

Servings: 6

Ingredients   Coconut oil - 1 Tbsp.

Cubed sweet potatoes – 2 cups

Yellow onion – 1, chopped

Garlic – 2 cloves, minced

Ground cumin - 2 tsps.

Buckwheat groats - ½ cup

Lentils – 1 cup, rinsed

Vegetable broth – 6 cups Salt - 1 tsp.

Ground black pepper – ½ tsp.

Chopped kale – 2 cups, stemmed

Directions: Melt the coconut oil in a pot.

Stir in the onion, sweet potatoes, garlic, and cumin. Sauté for 5 minutes. Add the lentils, buckwheat groats, vegetable broth, salt, and pepper. Bring to a boil. Reduce the heat to simmer and cover the pot. Cook for 15 minutes, or until the sweet potatoes, buckwheat, and lentils are tender. Remove the pot from the heat. Add the kale and stir to combine.

Cover the pot and let it sit for 5 minutes.

Serve.

Nutrition: Calories: 427

Fat: 7g Carb: 69g Protein: 24g

115.   Zucchini Patties

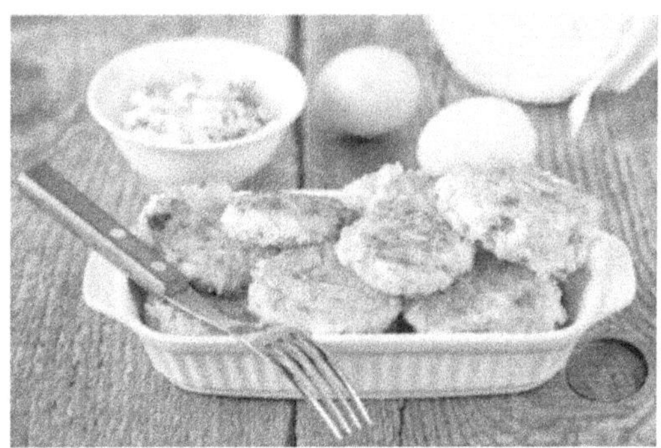

Preparations time: 15 minutes

Cooking time: 5 minutes

Servings: 2

Ingredients

Medium zucchinis – 2, shredded

Salt – 1 tsp. divided

Eggs – 2

Chickpea flour – 2 Tbsps.

Scallion – 1, chopped

Chopped fresh mint – 1 Tbsp.

Salt – ½ tsp.

Extra-virgin olive oil - 2 Tbsps.

Directions:

Place the shredded Zucchi in a strainer and sprinkle it with ½ tsp. salt. Set aside to drain.

In a bowl, beat together the chickpea flour, eggs, scallion, mint, and remaining ½ tsp. salt

Squeeze the zucchini to remove the liquid and add it to the egg mixture. Mix well.

Place a large skillet over medium heat and add the olive oil.

Drop the zucchini mixture by spoonfuls into the pan. Gently flatten the zucchini with the back of a spatula.

Cook until golden brown, about 2 to 3 minutes. Flip and cook for 2 minutes more.

Serve.

Nutrition:

Calories: 263 Cal Fat: 20 g

Carb: 16 g Protein: 10 g

116.   Shrimp Mix

Preparation Time: 10 minutes

Cooking time: 10 minutes

Servings: 4

Ingredients:

1 and ½ pounds shrimp, peeled and deveined

1 tablespoon essential organic olive oil

1 teaspoon sesame seeds

24 ounces broccoli florets

1 green onion, chopped

1 tablespoon balsamic vinegar

2 garlic cloves, minced

1 tablespoon ginger, grated

Directions:

In a bowl, mix oil with vinegar, garlic and ginger and whisk.

Transfer this to your pan, heat over medium heat, add shrimp, stir and cook for 3 minutes.

Add broccoli, stir, cook for 4 minutes more,

Add sesame seeds and green onions, toss, divide everything between plates and serve.

Enjoy!

Nutrition:

Calories: 265 Cal Fat: 2 g Fiber: 1 g

Carbs: 10 g Protein: 20 g

117.   Spinach and Lentils Stew

Preparation Time: 10 minutes

Cooking time: 23 minutes

Servings: 3

Ingredients: 1 teaspoon olive oil

1/3 cup brown lentils

1 teaspoon ginger, grated

4 garlic cloves, minced

1 green chili pepper, chopped

2 tomatoes, chopped

½ teaspoon turmeric powder

2 potatoes, cubed

A pinch of black pepper

¼ teaspoon cinnamon powder

1 cup low-sodium veggie stock

6 ounces spinach leaves

Directions:

Heat up a pot while using oil over medium heat, add chili pepper, ginger and garlic, stir and cook for 3 minutes. Add tomatoes, pepper, cinnamon, turmeric, lentils, potatoes, stock and spinach, stir and cook for 20 mins. Divide into bowls and serve. Enjoy!

Nutrition: Calories 220 Cal

Fat: 3 g Fiber: 11 g Carbs: 16 g

Protein: 11 g

118.   Sweet Potato Mix

Preparation Time: 10 minutes

Cooking time: 25 minutes

Servings: 4

Ingredients: 1 small yellow onion, chopped

1 tablespoon essential essential olive oil

2 garlic cloves, minced

4 sweet potatoes, chopped

1 red bell pepper, chopped

14 ounces canned tomatoes, chopped

2 teaspoons curry powder

A pinch of black pepper

2 tablespoons red curry paste

14 ounces coconut milk Juice of 3 limes

1 tablespoon cilantro, chopped

Directions:

Heat up a pot while using oil over medium heat, add onion, stir and cook for 5 minutes.

Add garlic, ginger, sweet potatoes, red bell pepper, tomatoes, curry powder, and black pepper, curry paste, coconut milk, lime juice and cilantro, stir and simmer over medium heat for 20 minutes. Divide into bowls and serve for lunch. Enjoy!

Nutrition: Calories 270 Cal

Fat: 7 g Fiber: 4 gCarbs: 12 gProtein: 7 g

119. Pea Stew

Preparation Time: 10 minutes

Cooking time: 25 minutes

Servings: 4

Ingredients: 1 carrot, cubed

1 yellow onion, chopped

1 and ½ tablespoons essential extra virgin olive oil

1 celery stick, chopped

5 garlic cloves, minced   2 cups yellow peas

1 and ½ teaspoons cumin, ground

1 teaspoon sweet paprika

¼ teaspoon chili powder

A pinch of black pepper

¼ teaspoon cinnamon powder

½ cup tomatoes, chopped

Juice of ½ lemon

1-quart low-sodium veggie stock

1 tablespoon chives, chopped

Directions:

Heat up a pot using the oil over medium heat, add carrots, onion and celery, stir and cook for 5-6 minutes. Add garlic, peas, cumin, paprika, chili powder, pepper, cinnamon, and tomatoes, fresh lemon juice, peas and stock, stir, bring to many simmer, cook over medium heat for twenty or so minutes, add chives, toss, divide into bowls and serve. Enjoy!

Nutrition: Calories: 272 Cal Fat: 6 g

Fiber: 7 g Carbs: 14 g Protein: 9 g

120.   Green Beans Stew

Preparation time: 10 minutes

Cooking time: 25 minutes

Servings: 4

Ingredients: 2 tablespoons essential olive oil

2 carrots, chopped 1 yellow onion, chopped

20 ounces green beans 2 garlic cloves, minced

7 ounces canned tomatoes, chopped

5 cups low-sodium veggie stock

A pinch of black pepper

1 tablespoon parsley, chopped

Directions:

Heat up a pot while using oil, over medium heat, add onion, stir and cook for 5 minutes.

Add carrots, green beans, garlic, tomatoes, black pepper and stock, stir, cover and simmer over medium heat for 25 approximately minutes. Add parsley, divide into bowls and serve for lunch.

Nutrition: Calories: 281 CalFat: 5 g

Fiber:1 g Carbs: 14 gProtein: 11 g

Dessert Recipes

121. Chickpeas Salad

Preparation time: 5 minutes

Cooking time: 0 minutes

Servings: 4

Ingredients:

2 cups canned chickpeas, drained and rinsed

1 tablespoon capers, chopped

2 tablespoons lime juice

2 tablespoons olive oil

4 spring onions, chopped

1 teaspoon chili powder

1 teaspoon cumin, ground

1 tablespoon parsley, chopped

A pinch of salt and black pepper

Directions:

In a bowl, combine the chickpeas with the capers and the other ingredients, toss and serve as a side salad.

Nutrition: Calories: 212 Cal

Fat: 4 g Fiber: 4 g Carbs: 12 g

Protein: 6 g

122. Quinoa and Beans

Preparation time: 10 minutes

Cooking time: 30 minutes

Servings: 4

Ingredients: 1 tablespoon olive oil

1 yellow onion, chopped 1 cup quinoa

½ cup canned black beans, drained and rinsed

2 cups chicken stock

2 garlic cloves, minced

Salt and black pepper to the taste

1 tablespoon cilantro, chopped

Directions:

Heat up a pan with the olive oil over medium heat, add the onion and the garlic and sauté for 5 minutes.

Add the quinoa and the other ingredients, toss, bring to a simmer and cook over medium heat for 25 minutes.

Divide everything between plates and serve.

Nutrition: Calories: 212 Cal Fat: 1 gFiber: 2 g Carbs: 2 g Protein: 1 g

123. Cucumber and Green Onions Salad

Preparation time: 5 minutes

Cooking Time: 0

Servings: 4

Ingredients:

2 tablespoons olive oil

2 cucumbers, sliced

4 spring onions, chopped

½ cup cilantro, chopped

½ cup lemon juice

Salt and black pepper to the taste

Directions:

In a salad bowl, combine the cucumbers with the spring onions and the other ingredients, toss and serve.

Nutrition:

Calories: 163 Cal

Fat: 1 g

Fiber: 2 g

Carbs: 7 g

Protein: 9 g

124. Barley and Kale

Preparation time: 5 minutes

Cooking time: 0 minutes

Servings: 4

Ingredients:

2 cups barley, cooked

1 cup baby kale

2 tablespoons almonds, chopped

2 tablespoons balsamic vinegar

1 tablespoon olive oil

1 tablespoon cilantro, chopped

Directions:

In a bowl, mix the barley with the kale, the almonds and the other ingredients, toss and serve as a side dish.

Nutrition:

Calories: 175 Cal

Fat: 3 g

Fiber: 3 g

Carbs: 5 g

Protein: 6 g

125. Herbed Mango Mix

Preparation time: 5 minutes

Cooking time: 0 minutes

Servings: 4

Ingredients:

2 mangos, peeled and chopped

2 spring onions, chopped

1 avocado, peeled, pitted and cubed

1 tablespoon olive oil

1 tablespoon chives, chopped

1 tablespoon oregano, chopped

1 tablespoon basil, chopped

2 tablespoons lemon juice

Salt and black pepper to the taste

Directions:

In a salad bowl, mix the mangos with the spring onions, the avocado and the other ingredients, toss and serve as a side dish.

Nutrition:

Calories: 200 Cal

Fat: 5 g

Fiber: 7 g

Carbs: 12 g

Protein: 3 g

126. Cabbage Slaw

Preparation time: 10 minutes

Cooking time: 0 minutes

Servings: 4

Ingredients:

2 cups green cabbage, shredded

1 carrot, grated

4 dates, chopped

2 tablespoons walnuts, chopped

1 tablespoon lemon juice

2 garlic cloves, minced

1 tablespoon apple cider vinegar

3 tablespoons olive oil

1 tablespoon parsley, chopped

A pinch of salt and black pepper

Directions:

In a bowl, combine the cabbage with the carrots, dates and the other ingredients, toss and serve as a side salad.

Nutrition:

Calories: 140 Cal

Fat :3 g

Fiber: 4 g

Carbs: 5 g

Protein: 14 g

127. Cucumber with Apples alad

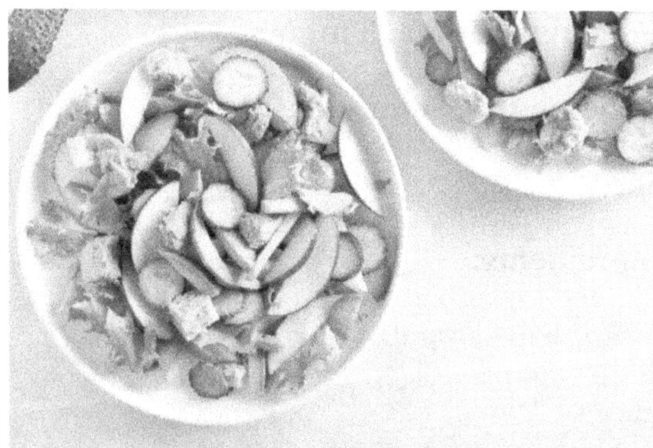

Preparation time: 5 minutes

Cooking time: 0 minutes

Servings: 4

Ingredients:

2 cucumbers, sliced

1 green apple, cored and cubed

3 spring onions, chopped

3 tablespoons olive oil

4 teaspoons orange juice

A pinch of salt and black pepper

1 tablespoon mint, chopped

1 tablespoon lemon juice

Directions:

In a bowl, mix the cucumbers with the apple, spring onions and the other ingredients, toss and serve as a side salad.

Nutrition: Calories 110 Cal Fat 0 Fiber 3 g

Carbs 6 g Protein 8 g

128. Parsley Avocado Mix

Preparation time: 5 minutes

Cooking time: 0 minutes

Servings: 4

Ingredients:

1 tablespoon olive oil

2 avocados, peeled, pitted and sliced

1 tablespoon parsley, chopped

1 tablespoon lemon juice

1 tablespoon lemon zest, grated

A pinch of salt and black pepper

Directions:

In a bowl, combine the avocados with the oil, the parsley and the other ingredients, toss and serve as a side dish.

Nutrition:

Calories 100 Cal

Fat: 0.5 g

Fiber: 1 g

Carbs: 5 g

Protein: 5 g

129.   Endives and Broccoli

Preparation time: 10 minutes

Cooking time: 20 minutes

Servings: 4

Ingredients:

2 endives, shredded

1 cup broccoli florets

2 tablespoons olive oil

1 tablespoon walnuts, chopped

1 tablespoon almonds, chopped

2 garlic cloves, minced

1 teaspoon rosemary, dried

1 teaspoon cumin, ground

1 teaspoon chili powder

Directions:

In a roasting pan, combine the endives with the broccoli and the other ingredients, toss and bake at 380 degrees F for 20 minutes.

Divide the mix between plates and serve.

Nutrition:

Calories: 139 Cal Fat: 9.8 g

Fiber: 9.3 g

Carbs: 11.9 g

Protein: 4.9 g

130.   Arugula Salad

Preparation time: 5 minutes

Cooking time: 0 minutes

Servings: 4

Ingredients:

2 cups baby arugula

Juice of 1 lime

½ cup cherry tomatoes, halved

1 tablespoon olive oil

1 tablespoon balsamic vinegar

A pinch of salt and black pepper

1 tablespoon chives, chopped

Directions:

In a salad bowl, mix the arugula with the lime juice, cherry tomatoes and the other ingredients, toss and serve.

Nutrition:

Calories: 190 Cal

Fat: 2 g

Fiber: 6 g

Carbs: 11 g

Protein: 7 g

Conclusion

It's clear that inflammation has both advantages and disadvantages to the body system. Its positive side involves healing joints, muscles, and body pains while its terrible side results from its good sides, which includes; causing heart attacks, stroke, soreness, and swelling, among others. Since a lot of prevention and treatment techniques have been discussed in the cookbook, everyone needs to understand their inflammation status.

Also, the anti-inflammation recipes compiled in this book are delicious, healthy, and easy to prepare. We have also simplified your shopping hassle by preparing a pantry list. You can begin by following our recipes and meal plans. After getting used, plan your dieting and modify your favorite dishes using anti-inflammatory ingredients. Note the number of servings before preparing any recipe for a balanced diet.

Inflammation of a body part is, in fact, the response given by the immune system to unfavorable stimuli like infections, damaged cells, and tissues, various pathogens, etc. Though this process is natural and quite harmless, it is something to worry about if the inflammation is persistent and chronic. In such cases it can do more harm than good and worsen the affected area.

The digestive tract or the gut is one of the most common sites of inflammation as a lot of pathogens enter the digestive system through the food we eat. Though the problem is not severe in most individuals, there are a lot of people who suffer from chronic inflammation. These recipes here will not only help to nullify the inflammation to a great extent but will also prevent further damage as well.

Inflammation has to be regarded as a serious condition, which can lead to devastating effects on your health. By reading this book, you have gained more knowledge about acute or chronic inflammation, and also about their causes. Although in some cases more research is required, most of us can agree that inflammatory conditions can be prevented and even reversed (in some cases). Probably you are not very convinced about the power of diets when it comes to health benefits, but by acknowledging the danger of inflammation and the benefits of anti-inflammatory foods, you should consider the meal plan presented in this book.

However, everyone should be cautious about their body health before taking vitamins, supplements, and the creams discussed to avoid more repercussions. Remember to seek your doctor's help before consuming them, and immediately you note any side effect after taking them.

ANTI INFLAMMATORY DIET COOKBOOK

The Book of Easy, Delicious and Tasty Recipes for Beginners, for Establishing New Eating Habits Based on Good Meals and Delicious Recipes

RIHANNA SMITH

TABLE OF CONTENCT

ANTI INFLAMMATORY DIET COOKBOOK

Introduction

What is Inflammation?

In the simplest terms, Inflammation is the process of how the body's immune system reacts whenever it detects the presence of a foreign entity inside the body or any form of injury. During an inflammatory response, White Blood Cells alongside a number of different substances tries to protect the body from further damage that might result from the contamination.

However, things change when this very action takes a turn for the worst.

Whenever you are dealing with something such as Arthritis, which is also related to chronic inflammation, the defense mechanism of the body seems to malfunction and trigger an inflammatory response even though there are no contamination.

Diseases that tend to do these are largely known as "Auto Immune" diseases and instead of protecting the body, the body's own auto-immune system starts to harm itself and damage the tissues

That being said, let's have a look at some of the main reasons of Inflammation.

What causes inflammation?

Various factors come into play when considering the reasons as to "What" causes inflammation in a human being. More often than not, a vast majority of the reasons tend to directly linked to poor Lifestyle choices, however, it should be noted that aging is a big factor here as well.

Some of the most crucial causes to know about include:

Aging

The natural process of aging contributes to Inflammation as well. As we age, few of our cells tend to regenerate and most of them start to die, leaving behind waste materials that tend to trigger inflammation.

Obesity and Inactivity

Excessive inactivity can and will often lead to obesity, which itself is a major cause of inflammation.

Adipose tissue, the layer of fat that is found right under our skin is actually responsible for much more than just keeping it warm.

It is a metabolically active layer that causes the body to change the body chemistry and is also affected by the body's other systems.

The fat layer contains a large number of white blood cells and greater number of fat (obviously).

However, the cell count is actually linked together. Meaning, the more fat there are, the greater number of white cells will be present.

These cells often tend to release pro-inflammatory substances that gradually contribute to the rise of inflammatory effects.

Diet

If we make a comparison, we would soon see that most of the causes of Inflammation are related to diet, so we are keeping this on the top of the list.

Harmful substances such as refined fats, animal products and refined carbohydrates tend to do a lot of damage in the long run.

It should be noted though that carbohydrates don't directly contribute to inflammation, but refined foods with higher concentration and fats are found to be naturally dense with inflammation causing substance that affect that gut and increases inflammation.

The types of fat that are consumed by an individual also plays a greater role here. Back in the early days when everything was simple, people used to stay on a diet that was very well balanced on both Omega 3 and Omega 6 fats. However, modern diets tend to have a very high concentration of Omega -6 fat as oppose to the Omega 3 fat, this increase the possibility of suffering from inflammation by 10-20%!

It's very important for the body to have a good supply of Omega-3 fatty acids because the Omega 6 and Omega 3, both compete for the same COX enzymes, which are needed to build large fatty molecules.

COX-2 enzyme in particular are essential for making inflammatory prostaglandins.

Too much of Omega-6 fatty acids will result in the domination of this enzyme and the body won't be able to utilize these enzymes anymore in conjunction with Omega-3 fats to reduce inflammation.

Nowadays fats are even chemically modified and this plays a greater role to inflammation as well. They are made to be more inexpensive, which results in the production of highly inflammatory products.

Stress

Cortisol is a hormone that is produced by adrenal glands and is used to manage the body's response to stress.

It helps to stimulate burst of energy and suppresses the action of pro-inflammatory substance.

This also helps to reduce stress by counter acting the effects of pro-inflammatory eicosanoids. However, if you stress too much, the amount of cortisol might increase to a dramatic level that will cause your immune cells to lose the sensitivity to this hormone and trigger inflammation.

Smoking

Exposure to various toxins such as cigarette smoke plays a great role in Inflammation. Either second hand or firsthand, inhaled tobacco tend to tends to extensively cripple the body's capacity to fight diseases by suppressing the production of white blood cells.

So, it's best to avoid smoking as much as possible.

Main Principles of the Anti-Inflammatory Diet

The anti-inflammatory diet is not merely a meal plan to maintain within a limited duration; additionally, it is not solely weight loss program as well.

Nevertheless, you can indeed lose weight by practicing it. Instead, the diet is a systematic way of choosing the right foods and preparing anti-inflammatory meals.

It derives its food selection and cooking processes on the scientific and medical knowledge of how your food intakes can help your body to attain and maintain optimum wellness. This natural dieting greatly influences the beneficial goals of inflammation.

The regimen provides you with a steady supply of energy, mainly sourced from the sufficient macronutrient consumptions. These intakes include dietary fibers and essential fatty acids. You will also have your ample share of vitamins and minerals from the micronutrient intakes.

Likewise, you can benefit more with the diet's protective phytonutrients. These are healthy and nourishing substances commonly derived from plants such as lycopene, lutein, and carotene.

People suffering from inflammatory diseases can reduce their inflammation and its side effects. They only need to radically change their diets. They can enhance the effect of taking prescribed medications with a proper nutrition program (anti-inflammatory diet).

Logically, if you intend to reduce inflammation, then consume less of the inflammatory foods. Instead, eat more and more of the anti-inflammatory foods.

Your regimen must provide for a healthy balance of macronutrients—fats, proteins, and carbohydrates—at each meal. Ensure also to meet your body's daily requirements for fibers, water, vitamins, and minerals.

Base your anti-inflammatory diet on nutrient-rich and whole foods containing antioxidants. These substances ably help to protect your cells from the destructive effects of oxidation.

In essence, antioxidants function by reducing the levels of free radicals. These are incredibly reactive compounds, which damage fats and proteins.

Free radicals also accelerate the progression of cardiovascular diseases, rheumatoid arthritis, cancer, radiation sickness, atherosclerosis, age-related illnesses, and many other health issues. Hence, avoid processed products, which are often dense with free radicals.

Generally, the natural design and function of the highly reactive molecules of free radicals are to assist metabolism. This biological process involves breaking down food compounds into smaller particles and disposing the absorbed nutrients into the blood to create energy for your body.

However, when you are unable to reduce or purge any intense reactions of these harmful free radicals, they can ultimately lead to inflammatory issues. You can only hold them in check through ingesting prescribed foods from the regimen.

Various Versions & Variations Of The Dietary Discipline: Replacement Regimens

The anti-inflammatory diet is a natural and nutritional regimen. As such, it encompasses most dietary plans.

The diet is relative to a wide range of recommended traditional and modern nutritional regimen. Its breadths and depths reflect the recommended food compositions.

The food elements include lots of fruits and vegetables, plant-based proteins (i.e., nuts and legumes), and fresh, organically grown herbs and spices. Whole grains and fatty fish are also among the regular staples.

If you were to account the macronutrient values, then the regimen inherently has limited calories (energy content of food), proteins, and saturated fats (solid fats). However, it is significantly rich in fibers or plant carbohydrates and trans-unsaturated fats (essential fatty acids).

Incidentally, these typical foods also form part of the core of food elements of several dietary disciplines. Three of these popular diets are the Mediterranean Diet, various types of Low-Carbohydrate Diets, and Vegan/Vegetarian Diets. Many nutritionists and dieticians consider these regimens as anti-inflammatory diets in nature.

Mediterranean Meals: The conception of the Mediterranean Diet was an inspiration of the time-honored dietary habits of people living within the Mediterranean region. The main feature of the diet is the high consumptions of olive oil, unrefined grains, legumes, fruits, and vegetables.

The regimen also includes moderate-to-high intakes of seafood and dairy products (often, yogurt and cheese). However, it restricts consuming non-fish and red meats. Its distinctive aspect emphasizes social celebrations of food with regulated intakes of wine.

Generally, it is a beneficial dietary plan rich in dietary fibers and monounsaturated fats while low in saturated fats. The Mediterranean Diet demonstrates to reduce inflammatory indicators like IL-6 and CRP.

Olive oil is the primary component of the diet that promotes good health. Studies insist that the regular consumptions of olive oil can lower mortality rates, neurodegeneration, and cardiovascular diseases. Additional studies also show that olive oil reduces the risks of cancer and several other chronic diseases.

Common Carb-Restricted Regimens: As its term implies, the dietary program emphasizes carbohydrate restriction. People often apply this typical regimen for the treatment or prevention of some chronic diseases.

These recurring health issues include high blood pressure and cardiovascular disease, gut fermentation and metabolic syndromes, and diabetes. It also reduces inflammation, especially for people who are obese.

The working principle of this diet entails limiting or replacing foods high in carbohydrates with foods that are rich in fats but moderate in proteins, as well as other foods low in carbs. The replaced food items are usually those easily digestible foods (i.e., pasta, bread, sugar, etc.), which have high glycemic indices (carb ratings that measure how quickly they raise blood sugar levels).

On one hand, these diets highly suggest consuming fatty foods with adequate protein contents. These food sources generally come from dairy, livestock, and poultry produce; nuts and seeds; and, seafood, particularly shellfish.

On the other hand, these diets recommended low-carb foods are those dark, green, and leafy vegetables. Low-carb diets also advise intakes of specific fruits, most preferably, berries.

The tolerable amounts of carb intakes vary with each specific low-carb regimen. Generally, a low-carb diet applies to meal plans that limit carb consumptions to less than 20% of one's recommended daily calorie intake.

For a steady and healthy dietary regimen, males require about 2,500 calories per day for healthy weight maintenance. Females need only to consume 2,000 calories each day. However, these figures may vary depending on age, body composition, and intensity levels of daily physical activities.

Similarly, low-carb diets may also refer to regimens that limit carb intakes to not more than the maximum recommended values. They use a rule of thumb for carb restrictions between 5% and 30% of your daily calorie intake.

The Ketogenic Diet is the chief proponent of this severe carb restriction regimen. The diet follows a regulated food consumption of 70% to 80% of calories from fats, 15% to 25% of calories from proteins, and 5% to 10% of calories from carbohydrates.

These caloric ratios fulfill the intents of inducing the body to enter into a state of ketosis. Ketosis is the occurrence of an excessive accumulation of ketones or fatty tissues in the bloodstream that the body cells use to burn for energy instead of carbohydrates.

The Atkins Diet also has a similar induction stage as the Ketogenic Diet. The only difference between these low-carb diets is the prescribed amounts of protein consumptions. The Atkins Diet proffers unlimited protein intakes along its 4-stage dietary plan.

The Paleo Diet is also a relatively low-carb regimen. It has a carb intake rating of 20% to 40% of calories from carbs.

The regimen distinctively summons the analogy of the eating patterns of our ancient ancestors who were initially hunter-gatherers. Thus, the diet mainly focuses on plant and animal foods low in carbs. Studies show that wild and organically grown plants contain fewer carbs and abundant in fiber compared to modern plant crops.

Vegan | Vegetarian Versions: Vegan and Vegetarian Diets carry the same wellness intent: to reduce inflammation. Engaging with the anti-inflammatory diet is like indulging with vegan protein sources or fatty fish instead of meat.

The principal staples of both Vegan and Vegetarian Diets are plant-based foods rich in vitamin K. These are mostly dark, green, and leafy veggies like broccoli, kale, and spinach. These leafy greens have long been heralded to help restrain inflammation.

Fresh fruits (i.e., blackberries, raspberries, etc.) are also essential food items of these plant-based regimens. The pigment that produces the specific colors for these fruits is a vital element in battling inflammation.

These versions and variations of the diet have already gained a foothold and a broader acceptance in today's society. Practitioners use them either as strategies to maintain good health or as medical nutrition therapies to manage their health issues. Nonetheless, most people commit themselves actively to these diets to seek protection against inflammatory conditions.

Summing it up, numerous studies have validated the countless health benefits of each of these regimens. For one, experts confirmed that vegetarians had increased levels of plasma amino acid (general health indicators associated with lower risks of heart disease and inflammation). In contrast, a recent study affirmed that consuming animal products increased the chances of acquiring chronic inflammation.

Gaining & Growing On Bountiful Benefits

Naturopaths, dietitians, nutritionists, and physicians are always inclined to prescribe the anti-inflammatory regimen. In all likelihood, they will endorse it as a complementary therapy for several health conditions aggravated by chronic inflammation.

Since it is a widely regarded healthy diet, it helps to lessen your chances of acquiring other health problems. That is, even if the regimen does not help with your current conditions.

The principal benefit of an anti-inflammatory diet is the reduction of inflammatory indicators in the blood. Foremost, it enhances blood sugar, triglyceride, and cholesterol levels.

The dietary regimen also boosts energy while improving your overall health and moods. In conclusion, strictly following an anti-inflammatory regimen and lifestyle, together with regular physical exercise and adequate sleep, can drastically reduce your risks of incurring many diseases, to wit:

- Active Hepatitis
- Alzheimer's disease
- Asthma
- Cancer, particularly Colorectal Cancer
- Chronic Sinusitis | Ulcerative Colitis
- Colitis
- Crohn's Disease
- Diabetes
- Eosinophilic Esophagitis
- Hashimoto's Disease
- Heart Diseases
- Inflammatory Bowel Syndromes (IBS)
- Lupus
- Metabolic Syndrome
- Obesity

- Peptic Ulcer
- Periodontitis
- Psoriasis
- Rheumatoid Arthritis
- Tuberculosis

The Anti-Inflammatory Diet Foods to Eat and Avoid

The anti-inflammatory diet can be restricted for specific types of foods. This is to ensure that you don't introduce things that might trigger inflammatory responses to your body. Although there are some types of foods that you should avoid with this particular diet, there is still a plethora of food groups that you are allowed to enjoy while following this diet.

Food groups	Anti-inflammation all-stars	Foods to avoid
Beans and legumes	Black-eyed peas, red beans, pinto beans, lentils, chickpeas, and black beans	NA
Fruits	Blueberries, blackberries, raspberries, strawberries, dark red grapes, cherries, coconut, avocado, and citrus fruits	NA
Allium vegetables	Onion, garlic, chives, shallots, leeks, green onions	NA
Vegetables	Cauliflower, broccoli, and cabbage. Also, dark leafy greens like mustard greens, collard greens, kale, lettuce, and spinach. Mushrooms, squash	NA
Nightshade vegetables	Tomatoes, bell peppers, eggplants, and potatoes	There is no scientific evidence that shows the nightshade group of vegetables have

		inflammatory properties. In fact, they are a nutritional powerhouse. Thus, if an individual is sensitive to nightshade food, then it is prudent to remove it from your diet.
Herbs and spices	Thyme, rosemary, cinnamon, basil, garlic, ginger, turmeric, chili peppers, paprika,	NA
Animal and fish products	Oily fish like herring, salmon, tuna, mackerel, and sardines. Lean meat	Avoid processed meats like sausages as they contain nitrites – a form of preservative that does little good to the body. Red meat like burgers and steaks
Recommended fats	Fats from coconut, avocado, olive oils. Fats from nuts like almonds, pine nuts, pistachios, and walnuts. Cocoa and chocolates	Fats found in fried foods; vegetable oil and soybean oil, margarine, shortening, and lard. Fats found in whole milk, butter—consider using low-fat dairy. Food laden with trans-fat such as processed foods should be avoided completely.
Recommended drinks	Green tea Red wine in moderation	Sugary drinks Excessive alcohol
Carbohydrates	Whole grains like unrefined grains, whole wheat bread, brown rice, oatmeal.	Refined carbs like white bread and pastries. French fries Artificial sugar should also be avoided.

The Science Behind the Anti-Inflammatory Diet

When your body needs to respond to an injury, it tends to mobilize an army of specialized cells to fend of the invading organism and toxins.

These cells prepare pathways for fighter cells to attack and completely engulf the attackers.

Once that has happened, another group of cells tend to signal to the body and let it know the fighter cells have accomplished their task and the body is allowed to stop the production of preparatory and fighter cells.

These results a sort of cleanup that clears up the leftover fighter cells from the battlefield and repairs any damage.

Simply put, there are two steps to this response:

Pro-Inflammatory

Anti-Inflammatory

Each cell involved in the pro stage builds on the work of the previous cells and helps to make the immune reaction stronger for any upcoming attack.

During the pro period, symptoms such as redness, swelling, itching are common.

The anti-inflammatory is the reverse of pro-inflammatory and it works to lower the effects of inflammation.

A variety of substances used to block inflammation are made from essential fatty acids, which the body isn't able to produce on its own.

These acids must be obtained through supplements or foods.

Two essential ones are Omega-3 and Omega-6.

Omega-6 tends to increase inflammation while Omega-3 helps to reduce it.

It should be noted that what I wrote above is a simplified version of the whole mechanism and there is a lot more to it.

There are various substances that play a deeper role in the whole infrastructure that allows the body to control its inflammatory mechanism.

Some of the crucial ones are:

Histamine: White blood cells near an injury tend to release a substance known as histamine. They increase the permeability of blood vessels around the wound that signals fighter cells and other substances to regulate an immune response and come to the sight of injury. Histamine also causes redness and swelling around the affected region and causes runny nose, rash, itchy eyes.

Cytokines: These are proteins that are activated by pro-inflammatory eicosanoids to signal fighter cells to gather at the injury site. They are responsible for diverting energy from the body to catalyst the healing process. Release of these substances tend to cause tiredness and decrease appetite.

C-Reactive Protein: Cytokines alongside other pro inflammatory eicosanoids are closely involved in the activation of a substance known as C-Reactive Protein. This particular organic compound produced by the liver responds to messages that are sent out by white blood cells. The C-Reactive proteins tend to bind the site of injury and act as a sort of surveillance unit that helps to identify the invading bodies.

Leukocytes: Several types of leukocytes (also known as white blood cells) are critical to the process of neutralizing invading substances. Neutrophils, for example, are small, agile and are able to first arrive at the scene of the crime to ingest small microbes. However, large substances such as macrophages as required to tackle a large number of microbes.

There are a few more, but the gist still remains the same. When your body starts to suffer from an uncontrolled inflammation attack, the action of these and similar substances tend to get out of control, which results in extremely uncomfortable situations.

Anti-Inflammatory Foods

An inflammatory response is caused by the activation of white blood cells in response to foreign entities in the body.

Whenever a molecule enters our bloodstream, our white blood cells immediately start to recognize that molecule as either belonging to the body or alien. If the molecule is foreign, it is tagged and removed to prevent it from causing any harm. The white blood cells also cause a series of processes, which are intended to minimize damage and contain pathogens.

For example, the chemicals released by the white blood cells often cause fluid to flow into the affected areas, therefore causing swelling. Likewise, redness often occurs due to increased blood flow (this helps white blood cells move to the appropriate place).

It is important to note that inflammation doesn't just affect the skin and joints, but it can also affect the internal organs. As you might expect, inflammation of the internal organs can cause serious health problems. Inflammation of the heart, for example, is called myocarditis and is associated with shortness of breath. Conversely, inflammation of the kidneys is also associated with high blood pressure and even outright kidney failure.

In some circumstances the inflammatory response arises due to a false positive, such as particular allergens, arthritis or an excessive intake of certain foods.

Inflammation is associated with redness, swollen warm joints, joint pain or stiffness and overall lack of malleability in the joints.

Inflammation has also been connected with a general reduction in well-being due to a myriad of flu-like symptoms such as pain, fatigue, headaches, fever and loss of appetite.

Therefore, if you find yourself suffering from any of these inflammatory symptoms then it can be useful to incorporate anti-inflammatory foods into your diet.

Current understanding is that there are dozens of potential sources of inflammation and just as many molecules that can help mediate both the causes and symptoms.

In particular, food scientists often record the presence of two proteins in the bloodstream (C-reactive protein & interluekin-6) as accurate indicators of the level of inflammation people suffer.

These two proteins are known to be controlled by omega-3 fatty acids, which are also known to have several other benefits (such as improving cognition).

Omega-3 fatty acids are present in several types of fish, including but not limited to

Salmon

Sardines

Tuna

Anchovies

Additionally, numerous nuts have omega-3, especially walnuts and almonds.

Inflammation is also thought to be reduced by a stronger and more efficient immune system. The exact mechanism by which a better immune system alleviates inflammatory response is not known, although there are a few hypotheses.

Namely, it is thought, that a more efficient immune system may manage problems faster, resulting in less time spent in an inflammatory response. Alternatively, a more productive immune system might produce fewer 'false positives' and react less severely to molecules, which are not genuinely harmful.

Regardless of the method, there is therefore reason to believe in a link between molecules that support the immune system (such as anti-oxidants) and lower levels of inflammation. The foods highest in anti-oxidants tend to be herbs & spices, although there are exceptions.

In particular the following foods are known to be especially potent;

Cloves

Ginger

Rosemary

Turmeric

Cinnamon

Allspice

Marjoram

Sage

Thyme

Italian Spice

Although you can supplement your meals with herbs and spices, their effect will be limited due to the small amount actually consumed. Therefore, it is also important to incorporate other foods, which are less powerful but can be eaten in greater quantities.

Many fruits & vegetables contain also contain high amounts of antioxidants and they can also feasibly be eaten in more meaningful quantities. Strong antioxidant choices include blueberries, blackberries, cherries, strawberries, spinach, kale & broccoli.

Additionally, foods high in monounsaturated fat should also be included in an anti-inflammatory diet. The exact reason why monounsaturated fat seems to have an anti-inflammatory effect is not known, although it has been suggested to be partially due to the presence of antioxidants and partially due to how monounsaturated fat promotes the absorption of vitamins & minerals (promoting overall bodily health).

Foods high in monosatured fat include nuts, seeds, olives, avocados and some types of vegetable oils. In particular, walnuts & almonds should make particularly prominent choices due to the fact that they also contain omega-3 and omega-6 fatty acids, which as previously mentioned, also have anti-inflammatory properties.

Other anti-inflammatory foods include most types of beans (such as kidney beans or butter beans). Beans are low in the glycaemic index, which categorizes foods by how quickly the carbohydrates within them are absorbed.

It is widely believed that inflammation may be partially due to excessive sugar and carbohydrate intake, foods with low glycaemic index values arguably have anti-inflammatory properties too.

Likewise, beans are high in fibre, which may promote overall gastrointestinal health and reduce intestinal inflammation. Fibre also lowers levels of the previously before-mentioned C-reactive protein (or CRP for short).

As a general rule of thumb, colorful fruits and vegetables are typically associated with both high levels of anti-oxidants as well as high levels of fiber, making them fantastic at lowering inflammation.

Moreover, several types of red wine can also be considered to be anti-inflammatory. Red wine, especially red wine originating from the Mediterranean and France, has been noted for its high levels of anti-oxidants.4

However, red wine also contains a molecule called Resveratrol, which is under research for its anti-inflammatory properties. With this being said, keeping alcohol intake within a reasonable level is obviously important for overall health.

Additionally, leafy greens (such as spinach, kale, collard greens & Swiss chard) are rich in multiple types of molecules that reduce inflammation.

Finally, consider adding tea (such as matcha tea & tulsi tea), blueberries, fermented foods, shiitake mushrooms & garlic.

To add to all of this, you might want to consider cutting some foods from your diet. Many of the usual unhealthy foods are suspected to increase inflammatory symptoms, such as processed foods, foods high in unhealthy fats and sodium.

Nonetheless, there are also some offenders you might not expect. The so-called nightshade branch of foods (which includes eggplant, tomatoes, peppers &) has been accused of exacerbating inflammation and arthritis. However, actual scientific support for this claim is rather sketchy.

To conclude, an anti-inflammatory diet would consist of a diet centered on the following foods;

Herbs & Spices

Fish

Nuts, Seeds, Avocado & Vegetable Oil

Fruit & Vegetables

Beans

Red Wine

Leafy Greens

The remainder of this eBook will provide you with numerous recipes high in these anti-inflammatory foods.

Breakfast Recipes

131. Morning Bowl

Preparation Time: 5 minutes

Cooking Time: 0

Servings: 1

Ingredients: 1 cup coconut milk

1 teaspoon raw honey

1 teaspoon walnuts; chopped.

1 teaspoon pistachios; chopped.

1 teaspoon almonds; chopped.

1 teaspoon pine nuts; raw

1 teaspoon pepitas; raw

2 teaspoons raspberries

1 teaspoon pecans; chopped.

1 teaspoon sunflower seeds; raw

Directions:

In a bowl, mix milk with honey and stir.

Add pecans, walnuts, almonds, pistachios, sunflower seeds, pine nuts and pepitas

Stir, top with raspberries and serve

Nutrition: Calories: 100 Cal Fat: 2 g

Fiber: 4 g Carbs: 5 g Protein: 6 g

132. Breakfast Stir Fry

Preparation Time: 20 Minutes

Cooking Time: 20 Minutes

Servings: 2

Ingredients:

1/2 pounds beef meat; minced

1 tablespoon tamari sauce

2 bell peppers; chopped.

2 teaspoons red chili flakes

1 teaspoon chili powder

1 tablespoon coconut oil

Salt and black pepper to the taste.

For the bok choy:

6 bunches bok choy; trimmed and chopped.

1 teaspoon ginger; grated

1-tablespoon coconut oil

Salt to the taste.

For the eggs:

2 eggs

1 tablespoon coconut oil

Directions:

Heat up a pan with 1 tablespoon coconut oil over medium high heat; add beef and bell peppers; stir and cook for 10 minutes

Add salt, pepper, tamari sauce, chili flakes and chili powder; stir, cook for 4 minutes more and take off heat.

Heat up another pan with 1 tablespoon oil over medium heat; add bok choy; stir and cook for 3 minutes

Add salt and ginger; stir, cook for 2 minutes more and take off heat.

Heat up the third pan with 1 tablespoon oil over medium heat; crack eggs and fry them.

Divide beef and bell peppers mix into 2 bowls

Divide bok choy and top with eggs

Nutrition:

Calories: 248 Cal

Fat: 14 g

Fiber: 4 g

Carbs: 10 g

Protein: 14 g

133.   Cereal Nibs

Preparation Time: 25 minutes

Cooking Time: 30 Minutes

 Servings: 4

Ingredients:

4 tablespoons hemp hearts

1/2 cup chia seeds

2 tablespoons coconut oil

1 tablespoon swerve

2 tablespoons cocoa nibs

1 tablespoon vanilla extract

1 tablespoon psyllium powder

1 cup water

Directions:

In a bowl, mix chia seeds with water; stir and leave aside for 5 minutes

Add hemp hearts, vanilla extract, psyllium powder, oil and swerve and stir well with your mixer.

Add cocoa nibs, and stir until you obtain a dough.

Divide dough into 2 pieces, shape into cylinder form, place on a lined baking sheet, flatten well, cover with a parchment paper, introduce in the oven at 285 degrees F and bake for 20 minutes

Remove the parchment paper and bake for 25 minutes more

Take cylinders out of the oven, leave aside to cool down and cut into small pieces

Serve in the morning with some almond milk.

Nutrition:

Calories: 245 Cal Fat: 12 g

Fiber: 12 g Carbs: 2 g Protein: 9 g

134. Chicken Muffins

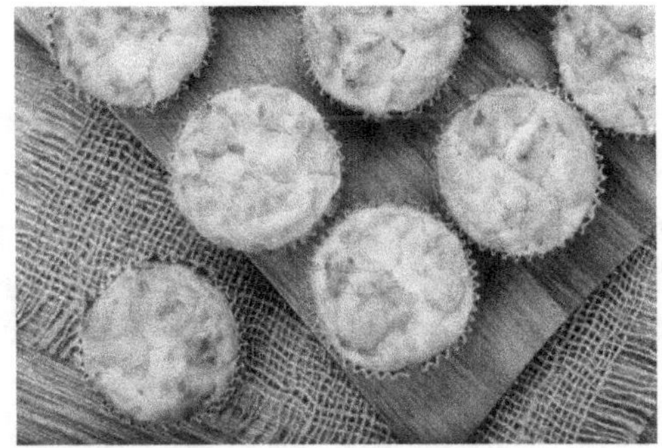

Preparation Time: 15 Minutes

Cooking Time: 55 Minutes

Servings: 3

Ingredients:

3/4-pound chicken breast; boneless

1/2 teaspoon garlic powder

2 tablespoons green onions; chopped.

3 tablespoons hot sauce mixed with 3 tablespoons melted coconut oil

6 eggs

Salt and black pepper to the taste.

Directions:

Season chicken breast with salt, pepper and garlic powder, place on a lined baking sheet and bake in the oven at 425 degrees F for 25 minutes

Transfer chicken breast to a bowl, shred with a fork and mix with half of the hot sauce and melted coconut oil.

Toss to coat and leave aside for now.

In a bowl, mix eggs with salt, pepper, green onions and the rest of the hot sauce mixed with oil and whisk very well.

Divide this mix into a muffin tray, top each with shredded chicken, introduce in the oven at 350 degrees F and bake for 30 minutes

Serve your muffins hot.

Nutrition:

Calories: 140 Cal

Fat: 8 g

Fiber: 1 g

Carbs: 2 g

Protein: 13 g

135.   Egg Porridge

Preparation Time: 14 minutes

Cooking Time: 0

Servings: 2

Ingredients:

2 eggs

2 tablespoons ghee; melted

1/3 cup heavy cream

1 tablespoon stevia

A pinch of cinnamon; ground

Directions:

In a bowl, mix eggs with stevia and heavy cream and whisk well.

Heat up a pan with the ghee over medium high heat; add egg mix and cook until they are done

Transfer to 2 bowls, sprinkle cinnamon on top and serve

Nutrition:

Calories: 340 Cal

Fat: 12 g Fiber: 10;

Carbs: 3 g

136.   Waffles

Preparation Time: 20 Minutes

Cooking Time: 10 Minutes

Servings: 5

Ingredients:

5 eggs; separated

4 ounces ghee; melted

3 tablespoons almond milk

1 teaspoon baking powder

4 tablespoons coconut flour

2 teaspoon vanilla

3 tablespoons stevia

Directions:

In a bowl, whisk egg white using your mixer.

In another bowl mix flour with stevia, baking powder and egg yolks and whisk well.

Add vanilla, ghee and milk and stir well again.

Add egg white and stir gently everything.

Pour some of the mix into your waffle maker and cook until it's golden.

Repeat with the rest of the batter and serve your waffles right away.

Nutrition:

Calories: 240 Cal Fat: 23 g

Fiber: 2 g Carbs: 4 g Protein: 7 g

137.   Quick Burrito

Preparation Time:10 Minutes

Cooking Time: 11 Minutes

Servings: 1

Ingredients: 1/4-pound beef meat; ground

1 teaspoon sweet paprika

1 teaspoon cumin; ground

1 teaspoon onion powder

1 small red onion; julienned 3 eggs

1 teaspoon coconut oil

1 teaspoon garlic powder

1 teaspoon cilantro; chopped.

Salt and black pepper to the taste.

Directions:

Heat up a pan over medium heat; add beef and brown for a few minutes

Add salt, pepper, cumin, garlic and onion powder and paprika; stir, cook for 4 minutes more and take off heat.

In a bowl, mix eggs with salt and pepper and whisk well. Heat up a pan with the oil over medium heat; add egg, spread evenly and cook for 6 minutes Transfer your egg burrito to a plate, divide beef mix, add onion and cilantro, roll and serve

Nutrition: Calories: 280 Cal Fat: 12 g

Fiber: 4 g Carbs: 7 g Protein: 14 g

138.   Poached Eggs

Preparation Time: 10 Minutes

Cooking Time 40 Minutes

Servings: 4

Ingredients: 3 tomatoes; chopped.

3 garlic cloves; minced

1 tablespoon ghee 1/4 teaspoon chili powder

1 tablespoon cilantro; chopped. 6 eggs

1 white onion; chopped.

1 red bell pepper; chopped.

1 teaspoon paprika

1 teaspoon cumin

1 Serrano pepper; chopped.

Salt and black pepper to the taste.

Directions:

Heat up a pan with the ghee over medium heat; add onion; stir and cook for 10 minutes

Add Serrano pepper and garlic; stir and cook for 1 minute

Add red bell pepper; stir and cook for 10 minutes

Add tomatoes, salt, pepper, chili powder, cumin and paprika; stir and cook for 10 minutes

Crack eggs into the pan, season them with salt and pepper, cover pan and cook for 6 minutes more

Sprinkle cilantro at the end and serve

Nutrition:

Calories: 300 Cal Fat: 12 g Fiber: 4 g

Carbs: 22 g Protein: 14 g

139. Pumpkin Pancakes

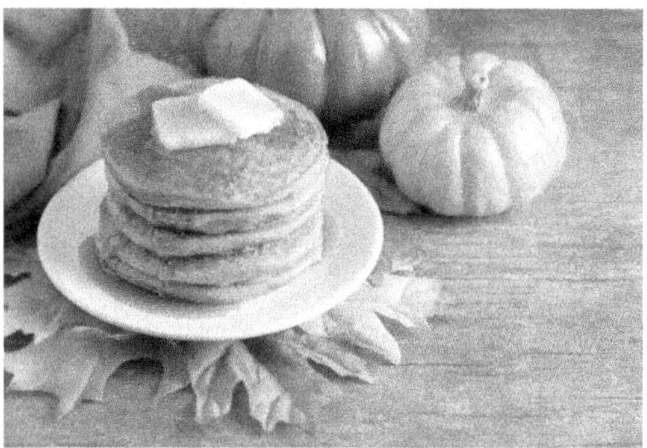

Preparation Time: 20 Minutes

Cooking Time: 5 Minutes

Servings: 6

Ingredients:

2 ounces hazelnut flour

2 ounces flax seeds; ground

1-ounce egg white protein

1 teaspoon coconut oil

1 tablespoon chai masala

1 teaspoon vanilla extract

1 teaspoon baking powder

1 cup coconut cream

1 tablespoon swerve

1/2 cup pumpkin puree

3 eggs

5 drops stevia

Directions:

In a bowl, mix flax seeds with hazelnut flour, egg white protein, baking powder and chai masala and stir.

In another bowl, mix coconut cream with vanilla extract, pumpkin puree, eggs, stevia and swerve and stir well.

Combine the 2 mixtures and stir well.

Heat up a pan with the oil over medium high heat; pour 1/6 of the batter, spread into a circle, cover, reduce heat to low, cook for 3 minutes on each side and transfer to a plate

Repeat with the rest of the batter and serve your pumpkin pancakes right away.

Nutrition:

Calories: 400 Cal

Fat: 23 g

Fiber: 4 g

Carbs: 5 g

Protein: 21 g

140.   Cauliflower and Chorizo

Preparation Time: 15 Minutes

Cooking Time: 40 Minutes

Servings: 4

Ingredients:

1 cauliflower head; florets separated

4 eggs; whisked

1/2 teaspoon garlic powder

2 tablespoons green onions; chopped.

1-pound chorizo; chopped.

12 ounces canned green chilies; chopped.

1 yellow onion; chopped.

Salt and black pepper to the taste.

Directions:

Heat up a pan over medium heat; add chorizo and onion; stir and brown for a few minutes

Add green chilies; stir, cook for a few minutes and take off heat.

In your food processor mix cauliflower with some salt and pepper and blend.

Transfer this to a bowl, add eggs, salt, pepper and garlic powder and whisk everything.

Add chorizo mix as well, whisk again and transfer everything to a greased baking dish.

Bake in the oven at 375 degrees F and bake for 40 minutes

Leave casserole to cool down for a few minutes, sprinkle green onions on top, slice and serve

Nutrition:

Calories: 350 Cal Fat: 12 g Fiber: 4 g

Carbs: 6 g Protein: 20 g

141.   No Cook Overnight Oats

Preparation Time: 5 Minutes

Cooking Time: 0

Servings: 1

Ingredients: 1 ½ c. low fat milk

5 whole almond pieces   1 tsp. chia seeds

2 tbsps. Oats   1 tsp. sunflower seeds

1 tbsp. Craisins

Directions:

In a jar or mason bottle with cap, mix all ingredients. Refrigerate overnight.

Enjoy for breakfast. Will keep in the fridge for up to 3 days.

Nutrition:

Calories: 271 Cal Fat:9.8 g Carbs:35.4 g

Protein:16.7 g Sugars:9 g

142.   Avocado Cup with Egg

Preparation Time: 5 Minutes

Cooking Time: 25 Minutes

Servings: 4

Ingredients:

4 tsps. parmesan cheese

1 chopped stalk scallion

4 dashes pepper

4 dashes paprika

2 ripe avocados

4 medium eggs

Directions:

Preheat oven to 375 0F.

Slice avocadoes in half and discard seed.

Slice the rounded portions of the avocado, to make it level and sit well on a baking sheet.

Place avocadoes on baking sheet and crack one egg in each hole of the avocado.

Season each egg evenly with pepper, and paprika.

Pop in the oven and bake for 25 minutes or until eggs are cooked to your liking.

Serve with a sprinkle of parmesan.

Nutrition: Calories: 206 Cal

Fat:15.4 g Carbs:11.3 g Protein:8.5 g

Sugars:0.4 g

143.   Mediterranean toast

Preparation Time: 10 Minutes

Cooking Time: 0

Servings: 2

Ingredients:

1 ½ tsp. reduced-fat crumbled feta

3 sliced Greek olives

¼ mashed avocado

1 slice good whole wheat bread

1 tbsp. roasted red pepper hummus

3 sliced cherry tomatoes

1 sliced hardboiled egg

Directions:

First, toast the bread and top it with ¼ mashed avocado and 1 tablespoon hummus.

Add the cherry tomatoes, olives, hardboiled egg, and feta.

To taste, season with salt and pepper.

Nutrition:

Calories: 333.7 Cal

Fat: 17 g,

Carbs:3 3.3 g

Protein: 16.3 g

Sugars: 1 g

144. Instant Banana Oatmeal

Preparation Time: 1 Minute

Cooking Time: 2 Minutes

Servings: 1

Ingredients:

1 mashed ripe banana

½ c. water

½ c. quick oats

Directions:

Measure the oats and water into a microwave-safe bowl and stir to combine.

Place bowl in microwave and heat on high for 2 minutes.

Remove bowl from microwave and stir in the mashed banana and enjoy.

Nutrition:

Calories: 243 Cal

Fat: 3 g

Carbs: 50 g

Protein: 6 g

Sugars: 20 g

145. Almond Butter-Banana Smoothie

Preparation Time: 5 Minutes

Cooking Time: 0

Servings: 1

Ingredients:

1 tbsp. almond butter

½ c. ice cubes

½ c. packed spinach

1 peeled and frozen medium banana

1 c. fat-free milk

Directions:

In a powerful blender, blend all ingredients until smooth and creamy.

Serve and enjoy.

Nutrition:

Calories: 293 Cal

Fat:9.8 g

Carbs:42.5 g

Protein:13.5 g

Sugars:12 g

146. Brown Sugar Cinnamon Oatmeal

Preparation Time: 1 Minute

Cooking Time: 3 Minutes

Servings: 4

Ingredients:

½ tsp. ground cinnamon

1 ½ tsps. pure vanilla extract

¼ c. light brown sugar

2 c. low-fat milk

1 1/3 c. quick oats

Directions:

Measure the milk and vanilla into a medium saucepan and bring to a boil over medium-high heat.

Once boiling, reduce heat to medium. Stir in oats, brown sugar, and cinnamon, and cook, stirring, 2–3 minutes.

Serve immediately, sprinkled with additional cinnamon if desired.

Nutrition:

Calories: 208 Cal

Fat:3 g

Carbs:38 g

Protein:8 g

Sugars:15 g

147. Buckwheat Pancakes with Vanilla Almond Milk

Preparation Time: 10 Minutes

Cooking Time: 4 Minutes

Servings: 1

Ingredients:

½ c. unsweetened vanilla almond milk

2-4 packets natural sweetener

1/8 tsp. salt

½ cup buckwheat flour

½ tsp. double-acting baking powder

Directions:

Prepare a nonstick pancake griddle and spray with the cooking spray, place over medium heat.

Whisk together the buckwheat flour, salt, baking powder, and stevia in a small bowl and stir in the almond milk after.

Onto the pan, scoop a large spoonful of batter, cook until bubbles no longer pop on the surface and the entire surface looks dry and (2-4 minutes). Flip and cook for another 2-4 minutes. Repeat with all the remaining batter.

Nutrition:

Calories: 240 Cal Fat:4.5 g

Carbs:2 g Protein:11 g Sugars:17 g

148. Tomato Bruschetta with Basil

Preparation Time: 10 Minutes

Cooking Time: 0

Servings: 8

Ingredients: ½ c. chopped basil

2 minced garlic cloves

1 tbsp. balsamic vinegar 2 tbsps. Olive oil

½ tsp. cracked black pepper

1 sliced whole wheat baguette

8 diced ripe Roma tomatoes

1 tsp. sea salt

Directions:

First, preheat the oven to 375 F.

In a bowl, dice the tomatoes, mix in balsamic vinegar, chopped basil, garlic, salt, pepper, and olive oil, set aside.

Slice the baguette into 16-18 slices and for about 10 minutes, place on a baking pan to bake.

Serve with warm bread slices and enjoy.

For leftovers, store in an airtight container and put in the fridge. Try putting them over grilled chicken, it is amazing!

Nutrition:

Calories: 57 Cal Fat:2.5 g

Carbs:7.9 g Protein:1.4 g Sugars:0.2 g

149. Sweet Corn Muffins

Preparation Time: 5 Minutes

Cooking Time: 15 Minutes

Servings: 1

Ingredients:

1 tbsp. sodium-free baking powder

¾ c. nondairy milk 1 tsp. pure vanilla extract

½ c. sugar 1 c. white whole-wheat flour

1 c. cornmeal   ½ c. canola oil

Directions:

Preheat the oven to 400°F. Line a 12-muffin tin with paper liners and set aside.

Place the cornmeal, flour, sugar, and baking powder into a mixing bowl and whisk well to combine.

Add the nondairy milk, oil, and vanilla and stir just until combined.

Divide the batter evenly between the muffin cups. Place muffin tin on middle rack in oven and bake for 15 minutes.

Remove from oven and place on a wire rack to cool.

Nutrition:

Calories: 203 Cal

Fat:9 g

Carbs:26 g Protein:3 g Sugars:9.5 g

150. Scrambled Eggs with Mushrooms and Spinach

Preparation Time: 5 Minutes

Cooking Time: 10 Minutes

Servings: 1

Ingredients:

2 egg whites

1 slice whole wheat toast

½ c. sliced fresh mushrooms

2 tbsps. Shredded fat free American cheese

Pepper

1 tsp. olive oil

1 c. chopped fresh spinach

1 whole egg

Directions:

On medium high fire, place a nonstick fry pan and add oil. Swirl oil to cover pan and heat for a minute.

Add spinach and mushrooms. Sauté until spinach is wilted, around 2-3 minutes.

Meanwhile, in a bowl whisk well egg, egg whites, and cheese. Season with pepper.

Pour egg mixture into pan and scramble until eggs are cooked through, around 3-4 minutes.

Serve and enjoy with a piece of whole wheat toast.

Nutrition:

Calories: 290.6 Cal

Fat:11.8 g

Carbs:21.8 g

Protein:24.3 g

Sugars:1.4 g

Meat and Poultry Recipes

151. Spicy Habanero and Ground Beef Dinner

Preparation Time: 10 Minutes

Cooking Time: 30 Minutes

Servings: 2

Ingredients: 1/2 teaspoon dried thyme

1/2 teaspoon ground black pepper

1/2 teaspoon dried basil

1 ½ pounds ground chuck

1 teaspoon habanero pepper, minced

1/2 teaspoon ground bay leaf

2 tablespoons tallow, at room temperature

2 ripe Roma tomatoes, crushed

2 shallots, chopped 1 teaspoon fennel seeds

2 garlic cloves, minced

1/4 teaspoon caraway seeds, ground

1/2 cup dry sherry wine

1/2 teaspoon paprika 1/2 teaspoon salt

For Ketogenic Tortillas:

A pinch of table salt 4 egg whites

A pinch of Swerve

1/3 teaspoon baking powder

1/4 cup coconut flour 6 tablespoons water

Directions:

Dissolve the tallow in a wok that is forehead over a normal high heat.

Following the above step, brown the ground chuck for 4 minutes, breaking it with a fork. Include all seasonings along with garlic, shallots, and habanero pepper. After that, keep on cooking for an additional 9 minutes.

Succeeding the above step, stir in the tomatoes and sherry. Then adjust the heat to medium-low, shut the lid, and let it simmer for a longer period of 20 minutes.

In the meantime, prepare the tortillas by mixing the coconut flour, eggs, and baking powder in a container. Add together the salt, water, and Swerve, then mix until everything is well included.

Foreheat a nonstick skillet with a moderate flame. Bake tortillas for a notable time on each side. Again, repeat until there is no more batter. Enjoy ground beef mixture.

Nutrition:

Calories: 361 Cal Protein: 29 g Fat: 21.9 g

Carbs: 6.4 g Sugar: 1.5 g

152. Meatballs with Roasted Peppers and Manchego

Preparation Time: 10 Minutes

Cooking Time 50 Minutes

Servings: 2

Ingredients:

2 leeks, chopped

2 ripe tomatoes, crushed

1 pound ground beef

1 teaspoon lemon thyme

3 garlic cloves

1 egg

3 tablespoons parmesan cheese, grated

1 ½ cups chicken broth

1/2 teaspoon fresh ginger, ground

4 bell peppers, deveined and chopped

2 chipotle peppers, deveined and minced

1/2 cup Manchego cheese, crumbled

Salt and freshly ground black pepper

Directions:

Heat- Broil the peppers for about 20 minutes while turning once or twice). Permit them to stand for about a minimum of 30 minutes to loosen the skin.

Skin the peppers; get rid of stems and seeds; slice chipotle peppers into equal parts and reserve.

In a mixing dish, merge the parmesan, leeks, egg, garlic, salt, pepper, and ground beef. Cook a heavy-bottomed skillet over moderately high heat.

Brown meatballs on all sides for about 10 minutes.

After the above step, make the tomato sauce. Cook the tomatoes, ginger, chicken broth, and lemon thyme in a pan that is preheated over medium-high heat; spice with salt and pepper to taste.

Enable it to boil, reduce the heat to medium. Add meatballs and let them simmer until they are completely cooked, careful stirring.

Serve meatballs with the tomato sauce and roasted peppers. Garnish with crumbled Manchego and serve!

Nutrition:

Calories: 348 Cal

Protein: 42.8 g

Fat: 13.7 g

Carbs: 5.9 g

Sugar: 2.7 g

153.   The Best Sloppy Joes Ever

Preparation Time: 10 minutes

Cooking Time: 20 Minutes

Servings: 6

Ingredients: 1 teaspoon deli mustard

Salt and ground pepper, to taste

1 ½ pounds ground chuck

2 teaspoons tallow, room temperature

2 shallots, finely chopped

1 tablespoon coconut vinegar

1 teaspoon chipotle powder

1 teaspoon celery seeds

1/2 cup pureed tomatoes

1 teaspoon garlic, minced

1 teaspoon cayenne pepper

Directions:

Dissolve 1 tablespoon of tallow in a heavy-bottomed skillet using a normal high flame.

After the above, sauté the shallots and garlic till they become tender and aromatic; reserve.

In the same skillet, dissolve another tablespoon of tallow. After that, brown ground chuck, crumbling with a spatula.

Include the vegetables back to the skillet; mix in the remaining ingredients. Set the heat to medium-low; simmer for 20 minutes; stirring every so often.

Enjoy over buns. Bon appétit!

Nutrition:

Calories: 313 Cal

Protein: 26.6 g

Fat: 20.6 g

Carbs: 3.5 g

Sugar: 0.3 g

154.   Grilled Rib Eye Steak

Preparation Time: 15 Minutes

Cooking Time: 5 Minutes

Servings: 6

Ingredients:

1 tablespoon Worcestershire sauce

2 tablespoons olive oil

2 tablespoons dry red wine

Celery salt and ground black pepper, to taste

1 tablespoon oyster sauce

2 garlic cloves, smashed

1 thyme sprig, chopped

2 rosemary sprigs, chopped

1 teaspoon dried sage, crushed

1/2 teaspoon chipotle powder

2 pounds rib-eye steaks

Directions:

In a mixing bowl, completely merge oyster sauce and garlic, Worcestershire sauce, thyme, rosemary, salt, sage, chipotle powder, pepper, wine and olive oil.

After that, marinate the rib eye steaks in your refrigerator overnight.

Preheat your grill that is previously lightly greased. Grill rib-eye steaks over direct heat for 4 to 5 minutes on each side for medium-rare. Bon appétit!

Nutrition:

Calories: 314 Cal

Protein: 48.2 g

Fat: 11.4 g

Carbs: 1 g

Sugar: 0.6 g

155.   Beef Sausage with Mayo Sauce

Preparation Time: 10 Minutes

Cooking Time: 5 Minutes

Servings: 4

Ingredients:

1 garlic clove, finely minced

2 tablespoons cilantro, minced

1/2 teaspoon dried marjoram

1/2 teaspoon salt

1/3 teaspoon red pepper flakes

1 tablespoon lard, at room temperature

1 red onion, chopped

1 tablespoon tomato puree

1-pound beef sausage, crumbled

For the Sauce:

1 ½ teaspoon mustard

1/4 cup mayonnaise

1 teaspoon cayenne pepper

A pinch of salt

Directions:

Dissolve the lard over medium-high heat. Include the onion and garlic and heat for 2 minutes or till they become tender and fragrant.

Stir in the beef and commence on cooking cook for about 3 minutes longer. Stir in the red pepper, salt, marjoram and cilantro; Heat for 1 additional minute.

After, make the sauce by whisking all the sauce ingredients. Enjoy over low-carb flat bread.

Nutrition:

Calories: 549 Cal Protein: 16.2 g

Fat: 49.3 g Carbs: 4.7 g

Sugar: 2.3 g

156. Slow Cooker Beef Chuck Roast

Preparation Time: 20 Minutes

Cooking Time: 6 Hours

Servings: 8

Ingredients:

1 large-sized white onion, cut into wedges

Salt and pepper to taste

2 rosemary springs 1 thyme sprig

2 tablespoons fresh parsley, chopped

2 tablespoons Worcestershire sauce

3 garlic cloves, minced

2 pounds beef chuck roast

1 cup Provolone, sliced

2 tablespoons olive oil

1/3 cup dry red wine 1/2 cup beef broth

Directions:

Include the beef, garlic, olive oil, onion, rosemary and thyme to your Crock pot.

After the above, include dry red wine, pepper, salt, Worcestershire sauce, beef broth.

Shut the lid and cook on High settings until meat is tender, duration of 6 hours.

Enjoy garnished with fresh parsley and sliced Provolone cheese. Bon appétit!

Nutrition: Calories:519 Cal Protein: 34.4 g

Fat: 39.6 g Carbs: 2.7 gSugar: 1.4 g

157. Finger-Lickin' Good Beef Brisket

Preparation Time: 1 Hour

Cooking Time: 2 Hours and 30 Minutes

Servings: 8

Ingredients: 2 garlic cloves, halved

1 teaspoon shallot powder

1/2 teaspoon freshly ground black pepper

1/4 cup dry red wine 1 teaspoon sea salt

1 tablespoon Dijon mustard

2 pounds beef brisket, trimmed

1 teaspoon dried marjoram

1 teaspoon dried rosemary

Directions:

Begin by preheating an oven to 3750F. Wipe the raw brisket with garlic and Dijon mustard. Now, Peform a dry rub by merging the remaining ingredients. Season the brisket on both sides using the rub. Transfer the wine into the pan. Lay the beef brisket in a baking pan. Roast in the oven for 1 hour. Reduce the temperature of the oven to 3000F; roast for an additional duration of 2 hours 30 minutes.

Now, slice the meat and enjoy with juice from the baking pan. Bon appétit!

Nutrition:

Calories: 219 Cal Protein: 34.6 g Fat: 7.2 g

Carbs: 0.6 g Sugar: 0.1 g

158. Winter Guinness Beef Stew

Preparation Time: 10 Minutes

Cooking Time: 50 Minutes

Servings: 6

Ingredients 1 ½ cups tomato puree

1 cup leeks, chopped

1 bay leaf 1 celery stalk, chopped

3 cups boiling water 1 cup Guinness beer

1/4 cup mint leaves, chopped, to serve

1 tablespoon beef bouillon granules

1 ½ pounds chuck shoulder, cut into bite-size cubes

1 ½ tablespoons avocado oil

1/2 teaspoon caraway seeds

Directions:

Apply heat to the oil in a stockpot over medium-high heat. Now, sauté chuck shoulder cubes till they are browned; reserve. Now, sauté the vegetables in pan drippings for about 8 minutes, stirring every so often. Add the remaining ingredients, leaving out formint leaves, and expose it to a rapid boil. After that, turn the heat to medium-low; allow it simmer for about 50 minutes. Scoop into individual bowls and serve garnished with mint leaves. Bon appétit!

159. Greek Prosciutto-Wrapped Meatloaf

Preparation Time: 10 Minutes

Cooking Time:50 Minutes

Servings: 8

Ingredients: 8 slices of prosciutto

2 teaspoons Greek seasoning blend

1/4 cup half-and-half

1/2-pound ground lamb

2 eggs, beaten 1 tablespoon Worcester sauce

3 teaspoons olive oil 2 pounds ground beef

2 shallots, finely chopped

6 ounces feta cheese, crumbled

1 tablespoon brown mustard

1/2 cup chopped Kalamata olives

Directions: Preheat your oven to a 3900F. Heat the oil in a cast-iron skillet that is fore heated using a medium flame. Sauté the shallot until it gets soft and lightly browned. In a large mixing container, completely merge the remaining ingredients, leaving out prosciutto. Add sautéed onion and stir well. Shape the merge substance into a meatloaf. Wrap the meatloaf in the slices of prosciutto and move it to a baking pan. Close it with a piece of aluminum foil. Bake for 40 minutes.

Nutrition: Calories: 444 Cal Protein: 66.3 g Fat: 14.2 g Carbs: 6.1 g Sugar: 2.7 g

Dispose of the foil and bake for an extra 10 to 13 minutes. Bon appétit!

Nutrition: Calories: 442 Cal Protein: 56.3 g Fat: 20.6 g Carbs: 4.9 g Sugar: 1 g

160. Greek-Style Cold Beef Salad

Preparation Time: 15 Minutes

Cooking Time: 3 Minutes

Servings: 6

Ingredients:

1 orange bell pepper, thinly sliced

1 green bell pepper, thinly sliced

1 tablespoon fresh lemon juice

Salt and ground black pepper, to your liking

1 cup grape tomatoes, halved

1 tablespoon soy sauce

1 ½ pounds beef rump steak

1/2 teaspoon dried oregano

1 head of butter lettuce, leaves separated

1 red onion, peeled and thinly sliced

2 cucumbers, thinly sliced

1/4 cup extra-virgin olive oil

Directions:

In a salad container, toss the onions, cucumbers, tomato, bell pepper, and butter lettuce leaves.

Fore heat a barbecue grill; heat the steak for 3 minutes per side. After that, thinly slice steak across the grain.

Include the slices of meat to the salad.

Prepare the dressing by whisking the oregano, salt, pepper, lemon juice, olive oil and soy sauce.

Dress the salad and enjoy well-chilled.

Nutrition:

Calories: 315 Protein: 37.5g

Fat: 13.8g Carbs: 6.4g Sugar: 2.4g

161. Slow Cooked Chicken Curry

Preparation Time: 10 Minutes

Cooking Time: 5 Hours

Servings: 4

Ingredients: 2 sweet potatoes, cubed

3 chicken breasts, boneless, skinless and chopped

1 red bell pepper, chopped

1 small yellow onion, chopped

2 cups coconut milk   2 cups chicken stock

1 teaspoon ground cumin

3 tablespoons curry powder

2 tablespoons chopped cilantro

Salt and cayenne pepper to the taste

Directions:

In your slow cooker, mix the chicken the sweet potatoes, bell pepper, onion, stock, milk, cumin, curry powder, salt and cayenne. Cover and cook on Low for 5 hours then divide into bowls, sprinkle the cilantro on top and serve.

Enjoy!

Nutrition:

Calories: 280 Cal Fat: 13 g

Fiber: 7 g Carbs: 8 g Protein: 15 g

162. Cumin Chicken Mix

Preparation Time: 2 Hours

Cooking Time: 25 Minutes

Servings: 4

Ingredients:

4 garlic cloves, minced

2 pounds chicken thighs, skinless and boneless

4 tablespoons extra-virgin olive oil

4 tablespoons chopped cilantro

2 tablespoons lime juice

A pinch of salt and black pepper

2 tablespoons olive oil

1 teaspoon cumin, ground

1 teaspoon red chili flakes

Lime wedges for serving

Directions:

In a bowl, whisk the olive oil with salt, pepper, cilantro, garlic, lime juice, cumin and chili flakes. Add the chicken, toss, cover and leave aside for 2 hours. Heat up a pan with the oil over medium-high heat, add chicken, cook for 3 minutes on each side and transfer to a baking dish. Cook in the oven at 375 degrees F for 20 minutes then divide between plates and serve with lime wedges on the side.

Enjoy!

Nutrition:

Calories: 200 Cal

Fat: 10 g Fiber: 1 g

Carbs: 12 g Protein: 24 g

163. Rosemary Chicken Thighs

Preparation Time: 10 Minutes

Cooking Time: 40 Minutes

Servings: 2

Ingredients:

14 ounces chicken thighs, bone-in

1 tablespoon lemon juice

1 teaspoon chili powder

A pinch of salt and black pepper

1 tablespoon fresh minced ginger

1 tablespoon olive oil

4 onions, chopped

2 rosemary springs, chopped

Directions:

In a bowl, mix chili powder with lemon juice and ginger. Add the chicken, rub it with this mix and then let sit for 10 minutes. Heat up a pan with the oil over medium-high heat, add the marinated chicken pieces and cook for 3 minutes on each side. Add rosemary, onions, salt and pepper. Reduce heat to medium, cover pan, cook for 25 minutes. Divide between plates and serve.

Enjoy!

Nutrition:

Calories 210 g

Fat 8 g

Fiber 9 g

Carbs 12 g

Protein 17 g

164.   Turkey Stew

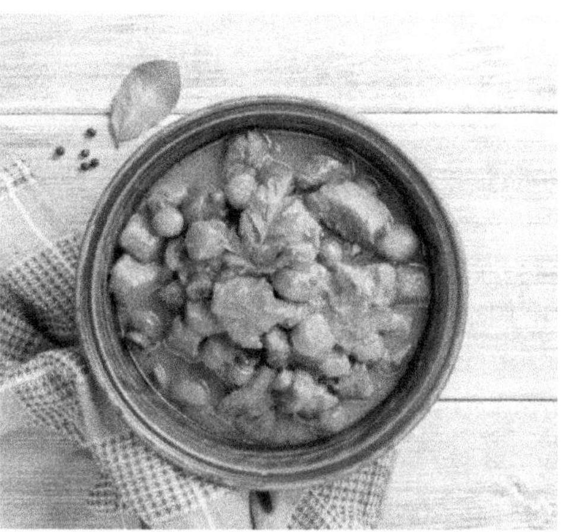

Preparation Time: 10 Minutes

Cooking Time: 1 Hour And 20 Minutes

Servings: 6

Ingredients:

3 teaspoons olive oil

1 green bell pepper, chopped

1 pound ground turkey meat

1 tablespoons garlic, minced

1 yellow onion, chopped

1 teaspoon ground ancho chilies

1 tablespoon chili powder

2 teaspoons ground cumin

8 ounces canned green chilies and juice, chopped

8 ounces tomato paste

15 ounces canned tomatoes, chopped

2 cups veggie stock

A pinch of salt and black pepper

Directions:

Heat up a pan with 2 teaspoons oil over medium heat, add turkey, stir, brown well on all sides and transfer to a pot. Heat up the pan with the rest of the oil over medium heat and add onion and green bell pepper. Stir and cook for 3 minutes. Add garlic, chili powder, ancho chili powder, salt, pepper and cumin, stir and cook for 2 more minutes. Transfer this to the pot with the turkey meat, add chilies and juice, tomato sauce, chopped tomatoes, stock, salt and pepper. Stir, bring to a boil, cover the pot and cook for 1 hour. Divide into bowls and serve.

Enjoy!

Nutrition:

Calories: 327

Fat: 8

Fiber: 13

Carbs: 24

Protein: 27

165. Chicken and Mushroom Salad

Preparation Time: 10 Minutes

Cooking Time: 0 Minutes

Servings: 4

Ingredients:

1 yellow onion, chopped

12 ounces canned mushrooms, drained and chopped

2 garlic cloves, minced

2 teaspoons chopped rosemary

3 cups chicken, already cooked and shredded

2 cups baby spinach

Salt and black pepper to the tastes

A splash of balsamic vinegar

A drizzle of olive oil

Directions:

In a bowl, mix the mushrooms with the chicken, onion, garlic, rosemary, spinach, salt, pepper, vinegar and oil, toss and serve.

Enjoy!

Nutrition:

Calories: 210 Cal Fat: 5 g

Fiber: 8 g Carbs: 15 g

Protein:11 g

166. Chicken Roast

Preparation Time: 10 Minutes

Cooking Time: 1 Hour And 10 Minutes

Servings: 4

Ingredients:

1 whole chicken

A pinch of salt and black pepper

2 tablespoons olive oil

2 green onions, chopped

1 cup chicken stock

2 teaspoons lemon juice

2 teaspoons chopped rosemary

Directions:

Place chicken in a roasting pan, add salt, pepper, oil, green onions, stock, lemon juice and rosemary. Toss the ingredients together, place in the oven and bake at 450 degrees F for 1 hour. Slice the meat, divide it between plates and serve with cooking juices drizzled on top.

Enjoy!

Nutrition:

Calories: 495 Cal Fat: 8 g

Fiber: 4 g Carbs: 10 g

Protein: 27 g

167. Ginger Chicken Thighs

Preparation Time: 12 Hours

Cooking Time: 1 Hour

Servings: 4

Ingredients:

8 chicken thighs, bone in and skin on

A pinch of sea salt and black pepper

1 tablespoon apple cider vinegar

3 tablespoons chopped onion

1 tablespoon fresh grated ginger

½ teaspoon dried thyme

¾ cup apple juice

½ cup maple syrup

Directions:

In a bowl, combine chicken thighs with salt, pepper, vinegar, onion, ginger, thyme, apple juice and maple syrup. Cover and keep in the fridge for 12 hours to marinate. Transfer this whole mix to a baking dish, cover dish, bake in the oven at 400 degrees F for 1 hour. Divide the meat and sauce between plates and serve.

Enjoy!

Nutrition: Calories 274

Fat 6 Fiber 8

Carbs 14 Protein 12

168.   Thai Chicken Thighs

Preparation Time: 10 Minutes

Cooking Time: 6 Hours And 10 Minutes

Servings: 6

Ingredients:

4 pounds chicken thighs, skin-on and bone-in

1 bunch green onions, chopped

½ cup Thai sweet chili sauce

Directions:

Heat up a pan over medium-high heat, add chicken thighs and brown them for 5 minutes on each side. Transfer the chicken to your slow cooker, add green onions and chili sauce, cover and cook on Low for 6 hours. Divide between plates and serve.

Enjoy!

Nutrition:

Calories: 260 Cal

Fat: 4 g

Fiber: 2 g

Carbs: 12 g

Protein: 14 g

169.   Chicken with Parsley Sauce

Preparation Time: 30 Minutes

Cooking Time: 40 Minutes

Servings: 6

Ingredients:

1 cup chopped parsley

1 teaspoon dried oregano

½ cup olive oil

¼ cup vegetable stock

4 garlic cloves

A pinch of salt and black pepper

12 chicken thighs

Directions:

In your food processor, mix parsley with oregano, garlic, salt, oil and the stock. Pulse well until smooth. In a bowl, mix the chicken with the parsley sauce and toss, cover and keep in the fridge for 30 minutes. Heat up your kitchen grill over medium heat and place the chicken pieces on the grill. Close the lid and cook for 20 minutes. Flip the chicken and cook for 20 minutes more. Divide between plates and serve with the parsley sauce on top.

Enjoy!

Nutrition:

Calories: 254 Cal Fat: 3 g Fiber: 3 g

Carbs: 7 g Protein: 12 g

170. Chicken and Lentil Casserole

Preparation Time: 10 Minutes

Cooking Time: 1 Hour And 40 Minutes

Servings: 8

Ingredients:

1½ cups green lentils

3 cups clean chicken stock

2-pound chicken breasts, skinless, boneless and cubed

A pinch of sea salt and cayenne pepper

3 teaspoons ground cumin

Cooking spray

5 garlic cloves, minced

1 yellow onion, chopped

2 red bell peppers, chopped

14 ounces canned tomatoes, chopped

2 cups corn

2 tablespoons chopped jalapeno pepper

1 tablespoon garlic powder

1 cup chopped parsley

Directions:

Put the stock in a pot, add a pinch of salt and the lentils. Stir, bring to a boil over medium heat, cover and simmer for 35 minutes. Heat up a pan with some cooking spray over medium-high heat and add the chicken, season with salt, cayenne pepper and 1 teaspoon cumin. Cook for 5 minutes on each side then transfer to a bowl. Heat up the pan again over medium heat, add bell peppers, garlic, onion, tomatoes, salt, cayenne and 1 teaspoon cumin. Stir, cook for 7 minutes and transfer to the bowl with the chicken. Drain the lentils, add them to the bowl with the meat and then add jalapeno pepper, garlic powder, the rest of the cumin, corn and parsley. Toss, transfer the whole mix to a baking dish and place in the oven at 350 degrees F and bake for 50 minutes. Divide between plates and serve.

Enjoy!

Nutrition:

Calories: 244

Fat: 11

Fiber: 4

Carbs: 10

Protein: 13

Seafood Recipes

171. Poached Halibut and Mushrooms

Preparation Time: 5 Minutes

Cooking Time: 30 Minutes

Servings: 8

Ingredients: 1/8 teaspoon sesame oil

2 pounds halibut, cut into bite-sized pieces

1 teaspoon fresh lemon juice

½ teaspoon soy sauce

4 cups mushrooms, sliced   ¼ cup water

Salt and pepper to taste   ¾ cup green onions

Directions:

Place a heavy bottomed pot on medium high fire.

Add all ingredients and mix well.

Cover and bring to a boil. Once boiling, lower fire to a simmer. Cook for 25 minutes.

Adjust seasoning to taste.

Serve and enjoy.

Nutrition:

Calories: 217 Cal Fat 15.8 g Carbs: 1.1 g

Protein: 16.5 g Fiber: 0.4 g

172. Halibut Stir Fry

Preparation Time: 5 Minutes

Cooking Time: 20 Minutes

Servings: 6

Ingredients: 2 pounds halibut fillets

2 tbsp olive oil   ½ cup fresh parsley

1 onion, sliced   2 stalks celery, chopped

2 tablespoons capers

4 cloves of garlic minced

Salt and pepper to taste

Directions:

Place a heavy bottomed pot on high fire and heat for 2 minutes. Add oil and heat for 2 more minutes.

Stir in garlic and onions. Sauté for 5 minutes. Add remaining ingredients, except for parsley and stir fry for 10 minutes or until fish is cooked.

Adjust seasoning to taste and serve with a sprinkle of parsley.

Nutrition:

Calories 331 Cal Fat 26 g Carbs 2 g

Protein 22 g Fiber 0.5 g

173. Steamed Garlic-Dill Halibut

Preparation Time: 5 Minutes

Cooking Time: 25 Minutes

Servings: 4

Ingredients:

1-pound halibut fillet

1 lemon, freshly squeezed

Salt and pepper to taste

1 teaspoon garlic powder

1 tablespoon dill weed, chopped

Directions:

Place a large pot on medium fire and fill up to 1.5-inches of water. Place a trivet inside pot.

In a baking dish that fits inside your large pot, add all ingredients and mix well. Cover dish with foil. Place the dish on top of the trivet inside the pot.

Cover pot and steam fish for 15 minutes.

Let fish rest for at least 10 minutes before removing from pot.

Serve and enjoy.

Nutrition:

Calories: 270 Cal

Fat: 6.5 g

Carbs: 3.9 g

Protein: 47.8 g Fiber: 2.1 g

174. Italian Halibut Chowder

Preparation Time: 5 Minutes

Cooking Time: 20 Minutes

Servings: 8

Ingredients:

2 tablespoons olive oil

1 onion, chopped

3 stalks of celery, chopped

3 cloves of garlic, minced

2 ½ pounds halibut steaks, cubed

1 red bell pepper, seeded and chopped

1 cup tomato juice

½ cup apple juice, organic and unsweetened

½ teaspoon dried basil

1/8 teaspoon dried thyme

Salt and pepper to taste

Directions:

Place a heavy bottomed pot on medium high fire and heat pot for 2 minutes. Add oil and heat for a minute.

Sauté the onion, celery and garlic until fragrant.

Stir in the halibut steaks and bell pepper. Sauté for 3 minutes.

Pour in the rest of the ingredients and mix well.

Cover and bring to a boil. Once boiling, lower fire to a simmer and simmer for 10 minutes.

Adjust seasoning to taste.

Serve and enjoy.

Nutrition:

Calories: 318 Cal Fat: 23g Carbs: 6g

Protein: 21g Fiber: 1g

175. Stuffed Salmon

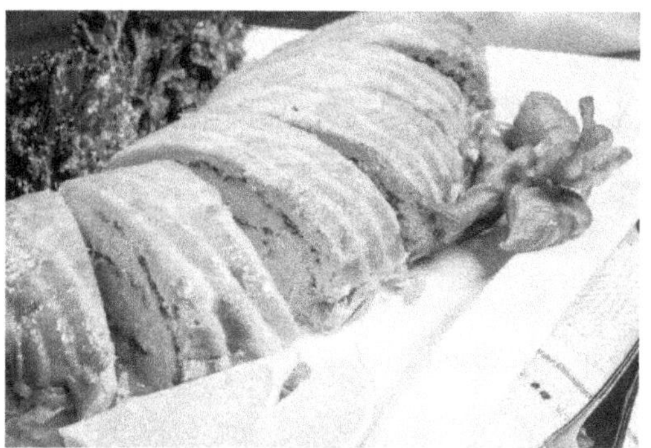

Preparation Time: 10 Minutes

Cooking Time: 20 Minutes

Servings: 2

Ingredients:

2 salmon fillets

4 teaspoons olive oil

5 ounces shrimp, peeled, deveined and chopped

6 mushrooms, chopped

3 green onions, chopped

2 cups baby spinach

¼ cup avocado mayonnaise

¼ teaspoon ground nutmeg

¼ cup chopped walnuts, toasted

A pinch of salt and black pepper

Directions:

Heat up a pan with half of the oil over medium-high heat, add mushrooms, onions, salt and pepper, stir and cook for 4 minutes. Add walnuts, spinach and shrimp then stir and cook for 4 minutes. Remove from the heat and mix with the nutmeg and mayo. Make an incision lengthwise in each salmon fillet then season with salt and pepper and stuff the salmon with the shrimp mix. Heat up a pan with the rest of the oil over medium-high heat, add stuffed salmon, skin side down and cook for 2 minutes. Reduce the heat, cover, cook the fish for 10 minutes. Divide between plates and serve.

Enjoy!

Nutrition:

Calories: 250 Cal

Fat: 10 g

Fiber: 3 g

Carbs: 7 g

Protein: 20 g

176. Mustard Crusted Salmon

Preparation Time: 10 Minutes

Cooking Time: 22 Minutes

Servings: 2

Ingredients:

2 salmon fillets, boneless

A pinch of salt and black pepper

4 tablespoons mustard

2 tablespoons coconut oil

Directions:

Season salmon with salt and pepper and brush it with the mustard on both sides. Heat up a pan with the oil over medium-high heat, place salmon flesh side down and cook for 3 minutes on each side. Transfer to a baking dish and place in the oven at 425 degrees F to bake for 15 minutes then serve with a side salad.

Enjoy!

Nutrition:

Calories 240 Cal

Fat 7 g

Fiber 6 g

Carbs 8 g

Protein 14 g

177. Dill Haddock

Preparation Time: 10 minutes

Cooking Time: 30 minutes

Servings: 4

Ingredients:

1-pound haddock fillets

3 teaspoons veggie stock

2 tablespoons lemon juice

Salt and black pepper to the taste

2 tablespoons mayonnaise

2 teaspoons chopped dill

A drizzle of olive oil

Directions:

Grease a baking dish with the oil, add the fish, also add stock mixed with lemon juice, salt, pepper, mayo and dill. Toss a bit and place in the oven at 350 degrees F to bake for 30 minutes. Divide between plates and serve.

Enjoy!

Nutrition:

Calories: 214

Fat: 12 Cal

Fiber: 4 g

Carbs: 7 g

Protein: 17 g

178.   Trout and Salsa

Preparation Time: 10 Minutes

Cooking Time: 16 Minutes

Servings: 2

Ingredients: 2 trout fillets, boneless

½ cup chopped yellow onion

4 teaspoons olive oil

1 teaspoon minced garlic

1 green bell pepper, chopped

½ cup canned tomato salsa

2 tablespoons kalamata olives, pitted and chopped

¼ cup chicken stock

A pinch of salt and black pepper

Directions:

Heat up a pan with 2 teaspoons oil over medium heat, add bell pepper and onion then stir and cook for 3 minutes. Add garlic, stock, olives and salsa, stir, cook for 5 minutes and transfer to a bowl. Heat up the pan again with the rest of the oil over medium heat, add fish, season with salt and pepper and cook for 2 minutes on each side. Transfer to a baking dish, pour the salsa over the fish and place in the oven to bake at 425 degrees F for 6 minutes. Divide between plates and serve.

Enjoy!

Nutrition: Calories: 200 Cal

Fat: 5 g Fiber: 6 g Carbs: 12 g Protein: 12 g

179.   Salmon Soup

Preparation Time: 10 Minutes

Cooking Time: 30 Minutes

Servings: 4

Ingredients:

1 red sweet bell pepper, chopped

2 green bell peppers, chopped

3 cups chicken stock

1 tablespoon olive oil

4 celery stick, chopped

1 brown onion, chopped

4 wild salmon fillets, skinless, boneless and cubed

A pinch of sea salt and black pepper

Directions:

Heat up a pot with the oil over medium-high heat, add the onion, stir and cook for 3 minutes. Add the red and green bell pepper, stir and cook for 3 minutes more. Add the celery, salmon, salt, pepper and the stock. Toss a bit then bring to a simmer, reduce heat to medium and cook for 20 minutes. Divide into bowls and serve.

Enjoy!

Nutrition:

Calories: 265 Cal Fat: 7 g

Fiber: 5 g Carbs: 15 g Protein: 16 g

180.   Shrimp Cakes

Preparation Time: 10 Minutes

Cooking Time: 10 Minutes

Servings: 24

Ingredients:

½ pound tiger shrimp, peeled, deveined and chopped

A pinch of sea salt and black pepper

2 tablespoons olive oil

½ pound ground pork

1 egg, whisked

2 tablespoons coconut flour

2 tablespoons chicken stock

1 teaspoon coconut aminos

1 green onion stalk, chopped

1 teaspoon fresh grated ginger

Directions:

In a bowl, mix the shrimp with the pork, salt, pepper, egg, stock, aminos, onion, ginger and flour. Stir well and shape medium cakes out of this mix. Heat up a pan with the oil over medium-high heat, add the cakes and cook for 5 minutes on each side. Divide between plates and serve with a side salad.

Enjoy!

Nutrition: Calories 281 Cal

Fat 8 g Fiber 7 g Carbs 19 g Protein 8 g

181.   Italian Calamari

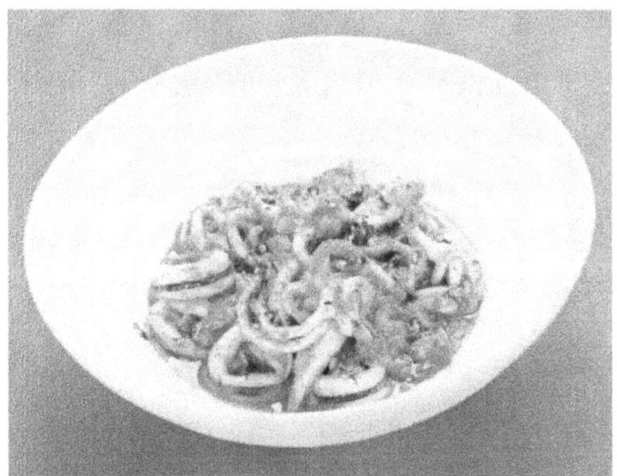

Preparation Time: 10 Minutes

Cooking Time: 30 Minutes

Servings: 6

Ingredients:

15 ounces canned tomatoes, chopped

1 ½ pounds calamari, cleaned, tentacles separated and cut into thin strips

1 garlic clove, minced

½ cup veggie stock

1 bunch chopped parsley

A pinch red pepper flakes

Juice of lemon

A drizzle of olive oil

A pinch of sea salt and black pepper

Directions:

Heat up a pan with the oil over medium-high heat, add the garlic and pepper flakes, stir and cook for 2-3 minutes. Add calamari, stir and cook for 3 minutes more. Add tomatoes, stock, lemon juice, salt and pepper, bring to a simmer then reduce heat to medium and cook for 25 minutes. Add the parsley, stir, divide into bowls and serve.

Enjoy!

Nutrition: Calories 228 Cal

Fat 2 g Fiber 4 g

Carbs 11 g Protein 39 g

182.   Chili Snapper

Preparation Time: 10 Minutes

Cooking Time: 20 Minutes

Servings: 2

Ingredients:

2 red snapper fillets, boneless and skinless

3 tablespoons chili paste

A pinch of sea salt and black pepper

1 tablespoon coconut aminos

1 garlic clove, minced

½ teaspoon fresh grated ginger

2 teaspoons sesame seeds, toasted

2 tablespoons olive oil

1 green onion, chopped

2 tablespoons chicken stock

Directions:

Heat up a pan with the oil over medium-high heat, add the ginger, onion and the garlic, stir and cook for 2 minutes. Add chili paste, aminos, salt, pepper and the stock, stir and cook for 3 minutes more. Add the fish fillets, toss gently and cook for 5-6 minutes on each side. Divide between plates, sprinkle sesame seeds on top and serve.

Enjoy!

Nutrition: Calories 261

Fat: 10 g Fiber: 7 g

Carbs: 15 g Protein:16 g

183.   Thai Cod

Preparation Time: 10 Minutes

Cooking Time: 10 Minutes

Servings: 2

Ingredients:

1 tablespoon coconut aminos

1 cup coconut milk

1 tablespoon Thai curry paste

A drizzle of olive oil

Zest of 1 lime

Juice of ½ lime

1 tablespoon fresh grated ginger

1 teaspoon garlic, minced

2 cod fillets, boneless

1 tablespoon chopped cilantro

Directions:

In a bowl, whisk the aminos with coconut cream, curry paste, lime zest and juice, ginger and garlic. Add the cod, toss to cover and set aside for 10 minutes to marinate. Heat up a pan with a drizzle of oil over medium heat, add the cod, cook for 5 minutes on each side, divide between plates and sprinkle cilantro on top then serve.

Enjoy!

Nutrition:

Calories: 271 Cal Fat 4 g

Fiber 6 g Carbs 14 g Protein 7 g

184.   Cod and Peas

Preparation Time: 10 Minutes

Cooking Time: 15 Minutes

Servings: 4

Ingredients:

10 ounces peas, blanched

1 tablespoon chopped parsley

A drizzle of olive oil

4 cod fillets, boneless

1 teaspoon dried oregano

2 ounces veggie stock

2 garlic cloves, minced

1 teaspoon smoked paprika

A pinch of sea salt and black pepper

Directions:

Put parsley, paprika, oregano, stock and garlic in your food processor and blend really well. Heat up a pan with the oil over medium-high heat, add the cod, season with salt and pepper and cook for 4 minutes on each side. Add the peas and the parsley, mix and cook for 5 minutes more. Divide everything between plates and serve.

Enjoy!

Nutrition:

Calories: 271 Cal Fat: 4 g

Fiber: 6 g Carbs: 14 g Protein: 15 g

185.   Salmon and Scallions

Preparation Time: 10 Minutes

Cooking Time: 20 Minutes

Servings: 4

Ingredients:

4 medium salmon fillets, boneless

4 scallions, chopped

2 tablespoons olive oil

Zest of 1 lemon

1 teaspoon white vinegar

¼ cup chopped dill

¼ cup chicken stock

A pinch of sea salt and black pepper

Directions:

Heat up a pan with half of the oil over medium-high heat, add the salmon, season with salt and pepper then cook for 6 minutes on each side and divide between plates. Heat up another pan with the rest of the oil over medium-high heat. Add scallions, stir and cook for 2 minutes. Add lemon zest, vinegar, dill, stock, salt and pepper. Stir and cook for 5 minutes more, pour over the salmon and serve.

Enjoy!

Nutrition:

Calories 300 Cal Fat: 4 g

Fiber: 8 g Carbs: 14 g Protein: 17 g

2 cups baby carrots

1 tablespoon lime juice

A pinch of sea salt and black pepper

Directions:

In a bowl, mix the cinnamon with half of the oil, salt and pepper then rub the salmon with this mix. Place the salmon on the preheated grill over medium-high heat, cook for 5 minutes on each side and divide between plates. Heat up a pan with the rest of the oil over medium-high heat and add the carrots, lime juice, salt and pepper. Toss and cook for 5-6 minutes then divide next to the salmon and serve.

Enjoy!

Nutrition:

Calories: 371

Fat: 26 Fiber: 2

Carbs: 6 Protein: 22

186.   Salmon and Carrots

Preparation Time: 10 Minutes

Cooking Time: 15 Minutes

Servings: 2

Ingredients:

1 tablespoon ground cinnamon

2 tablespoon olive oil

2 salmon fillets, bone-in

187. Chinese Mackerel

Preparation Time: 10 Minutes

Cooking Time: 30 Minutes

Servings: 4

Ingredients: 1 garlic clove, minced

1 shallot, chopped   1 cup chicken stock

2 pounds mackerel, skinless, boneless and cubed

1 small ginger piece, chopped

1 yellow onion, chopped

2 celery stalks, chopped

1 teaspoon hot mustard

1 tablespoon rice vinegar

A pinch of black pepper

A drizzle of olive oil

Directions:

Heat up a pan with the oil over medium-high heat, add the mackerel, season with black pepper and cook for 4 minutes. Add the garlic, shallot, onion, ginger and celery, toss and cook for 4 minutes more, flipping the fish as well. Add stock, mustard and vinegar, toss gently and cook for 20 minutes over medium heat. Divide into bowls and serve.

Enjoy!

Nutrition: Calories: 261 Cal Fat: 4 g

Fiber: 8 g Carbs: 14 g Protein: 7 g

188. Lemony Mackerel

Preparation Time: 10 Minutes

Cooking Time: 15 Minutes

Servings: 4

Ingredients:

Juice of 1 lemon

Zest of 1 lemon

4 mackerels

1 tablespoon minced chives

A pinch of sea salt and black pepper

2 tablespoons olive oil

Directions:

Heat up a pan with the oil over medium-high heat, add the mackerel and cook for 6 minutes on each side. Add the lemon zest, lemon juice, chives, salt and pepper then cook for 2 more minutes on each side. Divide everything between plates and serve.

Enjoy!

Nutrition:

Calories: 289 Cal

Fat :20 g

Fiber: 0 g

Carbs: 1 g

Protein: 21 g

189.   French Seafood Stew

Preparation Time: 10 Minutes

Cooking Time: 55 Minutes

Servings: 6

Ingredients: 1 fennel bulb, sliced

2 thyme springs, chopped

1 bay leaf

¾ cup olive oil

2 shallots, chopped

2 yellow onions, sliced

3 garlic cloves, minced

2 tomatoes, chopped

1-pound sea bass, skinless, boneless and cubed

1-pound snapper fillets, skinless, boneless and cubed

1-pound shrimp, peeled and deveined

A pinch of salt and black pepper

Directions:

Heat up a pot with the oil over medium-high heat, add shallot, onions and garlic and stir then cook for 4 minutes. Add fennel, thyme, tomatoes, bay leaf, salt and pepper, stir and cook for 5 minutes more. Add the fish and the shrimp, toss and cook for 5 minutes. Add water to cover everything and a little more salt and pepper then bring to a boil over medium heat, cover the pot and cook for 40 minutes stirring often. Remove the bay leaf then divide into bowls and serve.

Enjoy!

Nutrition:

Calories: 251 Cal

Fat: 4 g Fiber: 6 g

Carbs: 14 g Protein: 7 g

190. Scallops Stew

Preparation Time: 10 Minutes

Cooking Time: 20 Minutes

Servings: 4

Ingredients:

2 leeks, chopped

2 tablespoons olive oil

1 teaspoon chopped jalapeno

2 teaspoons chopped garlic

A pinch of salt and black pepper

¼ teaspoon ground cinnamon

1 carrot, chopped

1 teaspoon ground cumin

1½ cups chopped tomatoes

1 cup veggie stock

1-pound shrimp, peeled and deveined

1-pound sea scallops

2 tablespoons chopped cilantro

Directions:

Heat up a pot with the oil over medium heat, add garlic and leeks, stir and cook for 7 minutes. Add jalapeno, salt, pepper, cayenne, carrots, cinnamon and cumin, stir and cook for 5 more minutes. Add tomatoes, stock, shrimp and scallops, stir, cook for 6 more minutes then divide into bowls, sprinkle cilantro on top and serve.

Enjoy!

Nutrition:

Calories: 251 Cal

Fat :4 g

Fiber: 4 g

Carbs: 11 g

Protein: 17 g

Beans and Grains Recipes

191. Baked Beans and Rice

Preparation Time: 10 minutes

Cooking Time: 45 minutes

Servings 6

Ingredients:

1 ½ cups cooked brown rice

1 15-oz can no-salt added black beans, drained and rinsed

1 cup chopped poblano pepper

1 cup chopped red bell pepper

1 cup frozen yellow corn

1 cup shredded reduced fat Monterey Jack cheese

1 lb. skinless, boneless chicken breast cut into bite sized pieces

1 tbsp chili powder

1 tbsp cumin

2 14.5-oz cans no salt added tomatoes, diced or crushed

4 garlic cloves, crushed

Directions:

With cooking spray, grease a 3-quart shallow casserole and preheat oven to 400oF.

Spread cooked brown rice in bottom of casserole.

Layer chicken on top of brown rice.

Mix well garlic, seasonings, peppers, corn, beans and tomatoes in a medium bowl.

Evenly spread bean mixture on top of chicken.

Sprinkle cheese on top of beans and pop into the oven.

Bake for 45 minutes, remove from oven and serve.

Nutrition:

Calories 291

Fat 8g

Carbs 27g

Protein 27g

Fiber 5g

192.   Roasted Grain-Veggie Salad

Preparation Time: 15 minutes

Cooking Time: 45 minutes

Servings 6

Ingredients:

1 cup millet

1 cup quinoa

1/8 teaspoon curry powder (optional)

4 cups chicken stock or vegetable stock (more, as needed)

1/4 cup sun-dried tomatoes (dried in a package, not in oil)

1/2 cup boiling purified water

1/2 cup shredded zucchini

1/2 cup shredded yellow summer squash

1/4 cup minced red bell pepper

1/4 cup chopped scallions or green onions

Salt to taste

Directions:

Toast the millet and quinoa in a large saucepan set over low heat, stirring it constantly until it turns a light brown color, less than 1 minute.

Stir in the curry powder until it is blended in. Remove from heat and let cool for 5 minutes.

Add the chicken or vegetable stock and bring to a boil.

Reduce heat, cover, and simmer. Check after 20 minutes.

If the stock has boiled away, add a little more. Cook until the grains have absorbed all the liquid, about 25 minutes in all.

Meanwhile, soak the dried tomatoes in the boiling water for 15 minutes.

Drain them in a colander set over a bowl to reserve the liquid, then chop them.

Mix the tomatoes, reserved liquid, zucchini, yellow squash, red pepper, and scallions or green onions together in a small skillet set over low heat and cook until most of the liquid is absorbed.

Pour into the cooked grain and toss until everything is completely mixed together. Taste and add salt if you think it is needed.

Fluff with a fork and serve.

Nutrition:

Calories 153.9

Fat 6.2g

Carbs 22.7g

Protein 4.2g

Fiber 3.0g

193.   Tandoori Cauliflower-Rice Bowl

Preparation Time: 10 minutes

Cooking Time: 50 minutes

Servings 4

Ingredients:

2 tablespoons chopped fresh cilantro

1 English cucumber, seeded and diced

Lemon wedges, for serving

2 boneless, skinless chicken breasts (about 12 ounces total)

2 cups plain whole-fat yogurt

2 tablespoons lemon juice

3 teaspoons curry powder

2 teaspoons finely grated ginger

1 1/2 teaspoons finely grated garlic

Kosher salt

4 cups bite-size cauliflower florets (about 8 ounces)

1 tablespoon olive oil 2 ¾ cups water

2 cups basmati or other long-grain rice

1/4 cup tomato paste 4 wide strips lemon zest

Directions:

Slice chicken breasts into two thin slices.

In a bowl whisk well 2 tsp salt, ½ tsp grated garlic, 1 tsp grated ginger, 2 tsp curry powder,

1 tbsp lemon juice, and 1 cup yogurt. Divide yogurt mixture into two bowls. In one bowl, marinate chicken breast. In the other bowl, marinate cauliflower. Set aside for 15 minutes.

In large saucepan on medium high fire heat oil for 3 minutes.

Stir in rice and remaining garlic and ginger. Cook for a minute.

Stir in tomato paste and mix well. Add water, 1 tbsp salt, and lemon zest.

Bring to a boil. Once boiling, lower fire to a simmer, cover pan, and cook for 20 minutes.

Turn off fire, fluff rice, cover and let it rest for 5 minutes. Discard lemon zest.

In a medium bowl, mix well 1 tsp salt, 1 tbsp lemon juice, 1 cup yogurt, cucumber, 1 tbsp cilantro.

Preheat broiler and place rack on the topmost part of oven. Lightly grease baking sheets with cooking spray and lay marinated chicken on one sheet and on the other sheet evenly spread cauliflower.

Broil for 12 minutes.

Divide rice into four bowls. Top with ¼ of each of the cucumber sauce, cauliflower, and chicken. Garnish with remaining cilantro and lemon wedges.

Nutrition:

Calories 383 Fat 11g Carbs 44g

Protein 29g Fiber 6g,

194. Roasted Vegetables with Polenta

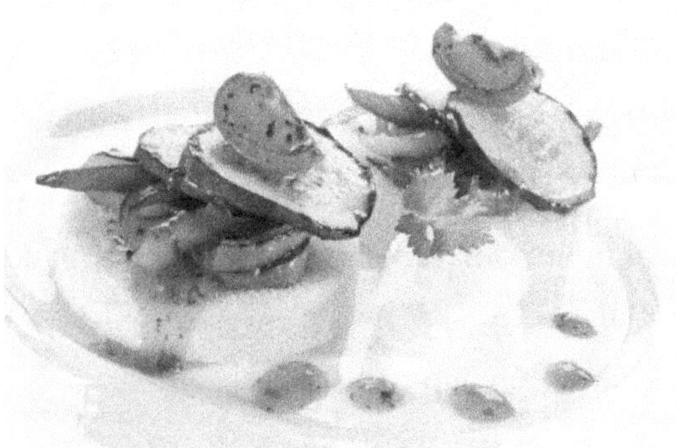

Preparation Time: 10 minutes

Cooking Time: 35 minutes

Servings 6

Ingredients:

2 tsp oregano

10 ripe olives, chopped

6 dry-packed sun-dried tomatoes, soaked in water to rehydrate, drained and chopped

2 plum or Roma tomatoes, sliced

10-oz frozen spinach, thawed

¼ tsp cracked black pepper

2 tsp trans-free margarine

1 ½ cups coarse polenta

6 cups water

2 tbsp + 1 tsp extra virgin olive oil

1 sweet red pepper, seeded, cored and cut into chunks

6 medium mushrooms, sliced

1 small green zucchini, cut into ¼-inch slices

1 small yellow zucchini, cut into ¼-inch slices

1 small eggplant, peeled and cut into ¼-inch slices

Directions:

Grease a baking sheet and a 12-inch circle baking dish, position oven rack 4-inches away from heat source and preheat broiler.

With 1 tbsp olive oil, brush red pepper, mushrooms, zucchini and eggplant. Place in prepared baking sheet in a single layer. Pop in the broiler and broil under low setting.

Turn and brush again with oil the veggies after 5 minutes. Continue broiling until veggies are slightly browned and tender.

Wash and drain spinach. Set aside.

Preheat oven to 350oF.

Bring water to a boil in a medium saucepan.

Whisk in polenta and lower fire to a simmer. For 5 minutes, cook and stir.

Once polenta no longer sticks to pan, add 1/8 tsp pepper and margarine. Mix well and turn off fire.

Evenly spread polenta on base of prepped baking dish. Brush tops with olive oil and for ten minutes bake in the oven.

When done, remove polenta from oven and keep warm.

With paper towels remove excess water from spinach. Layer spinach on top of polenta followed by sliced tomatoes, olives, sun-dried tomatoes, and roasted veggies. Season with remaining pepper and bake for another 10 minutes.

Remove from oven, cut into equal servings and enjoy.

Nutrition:

Calories 135

Fat 2g

Carbs 27g

Protein 5g

Fiber: 6g

195.   Cherries and Quinoa

Preparation Time: 5 Minutes

Cooking Time: 10 Minutes

Servings 1

Ingredients:

1 tsp honey – optional

¼ tsp ground cinnamon

½ tsp vanilla extract

½ cup dried unsweetened cherries

½ cup dry quinoa

1 cup water

Directions:

Wash quinoa in a bowl, by rubbing vigorously between your hands. Discard water and repeat rinsing two more times.

On medium high fire, place a medium nonstick skillet.

Add cinnamon, vanilla extract, cherries and quinoa.

Bring to a boil and stir occasionally.

Once boiling, slow fire to a simmer, cover skillet and cook until all water is absorbed and quinoa is tender, around 15 minutes.

Turn off fire and let it stand covered for 10 minutes more.

Transfer to a serving bowl and if using honey, pour and mix.

Serve and enjoy.

Nutrition:

Calories: 386 Cal

Fat: 5.3 g

Carbs: 72.12 g

Protein: 13.0 g

Fiber: 7.7 g

196. Granola from Quinoa and Buckwheat

Preparation Time: 5 Minutes

Cooking Time: 45 Minutes

Servings 6

Ingredients: ½ cup old fashioned oats

½ cup dried unsweetened cranberries

1 cup cooked quinoa 1 cup buckwheat groats

¼ tsp ground ginger

¼ tsp ground cinnamon

1 tsp vanilla extract

1 tbsp liquid coconut oil

3 tbsp honey

Directions:

Grease a baking sheet and preheat oven to 325oF. In a large bowl, mix well oats, quinoa and buckwheat.

In a small bowl, stir well honey, coconut oil, vanilla, cinnamon, and ginger. Pour into bowl of oats and mix well. In an even layer, spread the mixture on baking sheet.

Pop into the oven and bake until grains begin to brown around 40 to 45 minutes. Remove from oven and stir in cranberries. Let it cool before serving or storing.

Nutrition: Calories: 146 Cal Fat: 4 g

Protein: 4 g Fiber: 3 g

197. Trout 'n Cannellini Tartine

Preparation Time: 10minutes

Cooking Time: 0 Minutes

Servings: 4

Ingredients: Dill sprigs – for garnish

4 large whole grain bread, toasted

1 tsp chopped fresh dill 2 tsp minced onion

1 stalk celery, finely chopped

½ 15-oz can cannellini beans

½ cup diced roasted red peppers

2 tbsp capers, rinsed and drained

¾ lb. smoked trout, flaked into bite-sized pieces

Pinch of sugar 1 tsp Dijon mustard

1 tbsp extra virgin olive oil

2 tbsp freshly squeezed lemon juice

Directions:

Mix sugar, mustard, olive oil and lemon juice in a big bowl. Add the rest of the ingredients except for toasted bread.

Toss to mix well.

Evenly divide fish mixture on top of bread slices and garnish with dill sprigs.

Serve and enjoy.

Nutrition: Calories: 253 Cal Fat: 9 g

Carbs: 17 g Protein: 25 g Fiber: 4 g

198.   Brussels Sprouts 'n White Bean Medley

Prepration Time: 10 Minutes

Cooking Time: 20 Minutes

Servings: 4

Ingredients: Pepper to taste

6 garlic cloves, smashed, peeled, and minced

4 ½ cups Brussels sprouts, cleaned and sliced in half

3tbsp lemon juice

3 medium onions, peeled and sliced

3 cans white beans, drained and rinsed

1 tbsp olive oil 1 tsp salt

Directions:

Place a saucepan on medium high fire and heat for 2 minutes.

Add oil and heat for a minute.

Sauté garlic and onions for 3 minutes.

Stir in Brussels Sprouts and sauté for 5 minutes.

Stir in white beans and sauté for 5 minutes.

Season with pepper and salt.

Nutrition:

Calories 329 Fat 5g

Carbs 55g Protein 18g

Fiber 16g

199.   Quinoa and Kidney Beans Pilaf

Preparation Time: 10 Minutes

Cooking Time: 40 Minutes

Servings: 4

Ingredients:

¼ teaspoon red pepper flakes

¼ teaspoon smoked paprika

½ teaspoon cumin

½ teaspoon sea salt

1 3/4 cups water

1 cup quinoa, uncooked

1 large clove garlic minced

1 small red bell pepper finely diced

1 small red onion finely diced

1 tablespoon tomato paste

1 15-ounce can kidney beans rinsed and drained

1 tsp olive oil

Directions:

Place a nonstick pot on medium high fire and heat oil for 2 minutes.

Stir in peppers and onion. Sauté for 5 minutes.

Add tomato paste, red pepper flakes, salt, paprika, cumin, and garlic. Sauté for 2 minutes.

Stir in quinoa and mix well. Sauté for 2 minutes.

Add water and beans. Mix well. Cover and simmer for 20 minutes or until liquid is fully absorbed.

Turn off fire and fluff quinoa. Let it sit for 5 minutes more while uncovered.

Serve and enjoy.

Nutrition:

Calories: 317 Cal Fat: 5 g

Carbs: 54 g Protein: 15 g Fiber: 10 g

Kidney Bean Salad with Vinaigrette

Preparation Time: 10 Minutes

Cooking Time: 10 Minutes

Servings: 4

Ingredients:

1 15-oz. can kidney beans, drained and rinsed

1/2 English cucumbers, chopped

1 Medium-sized heirloom tomato, chopped

1 bunch fresh cilantro, stems removed, chopped (about 1 1/4 cup)

1 red onion, chopped (about 1 cup)

Cilantro-Dijon Vinaigrette Ingredients:

1 large lime or lemon, juiced

3 tbsp extra virgin olive oil

1 tsp Dijon mustard

½ tsp fresh garlic paste, or finely chopped garlic

1 tsp sumac

Salt and pepper, to taste

Directions:

In a small bowl, whisk well all vinaigrette ingredients.

In a salad bowl, combine cilantro chopped veggies, and kidney beans.

Add vinaigrette to salad and toss well to mix.

For 30 minutes allow for flavors to mix and set in the fridge.

Mix and adjust seasoning if needed before serving.

Nutrition:

Calories: 250 Cal

Fat: 11 g

Carbs: 30 g

Protein: 10 g

Fiber: 8 g

Kidney Beans in Mexican Rice

Preparation Time: 10 Minutes

Cooking Time: 25 Minutes

Servings: 6

Ingredients:

2 tablespoons olive oil

2 cups julienned bell peppers

1 cup crushed tomatoes

1 cup corn kernels

2 tablespoons green chilies

1 tablespoon oregano

1 to 2 teaspoons chili powder to taste

3 cups cooked brown rice

Salt to taste

1/2 cup shredded purple cabbage

1 1/2 cups mixed veggies

1 1/2 teaspoons cumin

1/4 to 1/2 teaspoon liquid smoke to taste

1/4 cup minced onion

1 14.5 ounces can diced tomatoes

1 15.5 ounce can kidney beans

Directions

Place a large saucepan on medium high fire and heat for 2 minutes.

Add oil and heat for another 2 minutes. Stir in onions and sauté for 4 minutes.

Add cabbage and bell peppers, sauté for 3 minutes.

Stir in liquid smoke, chili powder, cumin, oregano, green chiles, corn, kidney beans, tomatoes, and mixed vegetables. Mix well.

Cover and cook for 9 minutes, mixing occasionally.

Stir in the cooked rice and lower fire to medium low. Mix rice well until colored red.

Adjust seasoning to taste, serve and enjoy one rice is heated through.

Nutrition:

Calories: 320 Cal

Fat: 8 g

Carbs: 55 g

Protein: 11 g

200.   Green Hummus

Preparation Time: 10 Minutes

Cooking Time: 10 Minutes

Servings: 8

Ingredients:

¼ cup fresh lemon juice (about 1 large lemon's worth)

¼ cup roughly chopped, loosely packed fresh tarragon or basil - ¼ cup tahini

½ cup roughly chopped, loosely packed fresh parsley

½ teaspoon salt, more to taste

1 large garlic clove, roughly chopped

1 to 2 tablespoons water, optional

2 tablespoons olive oil, plus more for serving

2 to 3 tablespoons roughly chopped fresh chives or green onion

Garnish with extra olive oil and a sprinkling of chopped fresh herbs

One (15-ounce) can of chickpeas, also called garbanzo beans, drained and rinsed

Directions: Place al ingredients in a blender and puree until smooth and creamy. Transfer to a bowl and adjust seasoning if needed. Serve with pita chips.

Nutrition: Calories: 139 Cal Fat: 10 g

Carbs: 10 gProtein: 4 gFiber: 3 g

201.   Parsley 'n Lemon Kidney Beans

Preparation Time: 10 Minutes

Cooking Time: 0

Servings: 6

Ingredients: 3 cloves garlic, pressed or minced - ¼ cup lemon juice (about 1 ½ lemons)

¼ cup olive oil ¾ cup chopped fresh parsley

¾ teaspoon salt 1 small red onion, diced

1 can (15 ounces) chickpeas, rinsed and drained

1 medium cucumber, peeled, seeded and diced

2 cans (15 ounces each) red kidney beans, rinsed and drained

2 stalks celery, sliced in half or thirds lengthwise and chopped

2 tablespoons chopped fresh dill or mint

Small pinch red pepper flakes

Directions: Whisk well in a small bowl the pepper flakes, salt, garlic, and lemon juice until emulsified. In a serving bowl, combine the prepared kidney beans, chickpeas, onion, celery, cucumber, parsley and dill (or mint). Drizzle salad with the dressing and toss well to coat. Serve and enjoy.

Nutrition: Calories 345 Fat 11g

Carbs 47g Protein 16g Fiber 15g

202. Moroccan Salad

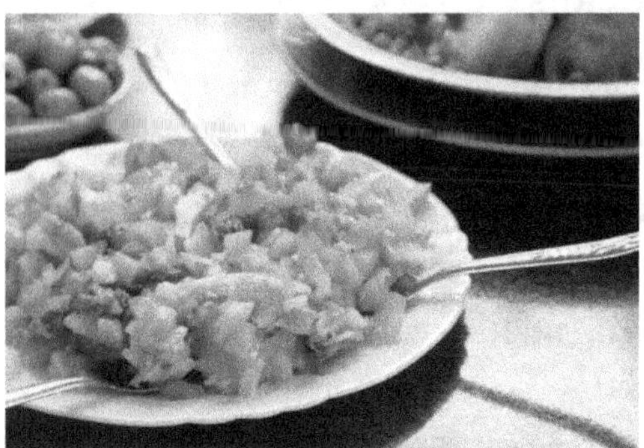

Preparation Time: 10 Minutes

Cooking Time: 0

Servings: 10

Ingredients:

¼ cup lemon juice

¼ teaspoon ground cinnamon

½ cup chopped fresh mint

½ cup extra-virgin olive oil

1 15-ounce can chickpeas, rinsed

1 cup finely diced carrot

1 small clove garlic, peeled and minced

1 teaspoon kosher salt, divided

1½ cups chopped fresh parsley

2 15-ounce cans dark red kidney beans, rinsed

2 tablespoons ground cumin

Directions:

In a salad bowl, whisk well lemon juice, cinnamon, olive oil, garlic, salt, parsley, and cumin.

Stir in remaining ingredients and toss well to coat in the dressing.

Serve and enjoy.

Nutrition:

Calories: 196 Cal Fat: 6 g

Carbs: 27 g Protein: 9 g

Fiber: 9 g

203. Blue Cheese 'n Pears on Grains Salad

Preparation Time: 10 minutes

Cooking Time: 40 minutes

Servings 4

Ingredients:

¼ cup thinly sliced scallions

½ cup millet, rinsed

½ cup quinoa, rinsed

1 ½ tsp olive oil

1 Bartlett pear, cored and diced

1/8 tsp ground black pepper

2 cloves garlic, minced

2 oz blue cheese

2 tbsp fresh lemon juice

2 tsp dried rosemary

4 4-oz boneless, skinless chicken breasts

6 oz baby spinach

olive oil cooking spray

Dressing Ingredients:

¼ cup fresh raspberries

1 tbsp pure maple syrup

1 tsp fresh thyme leaf

2 tbsp grainy mustard

6 tbsp balsamic vinegar

Directions:

Bring millet, quinoa, and 2 ¼ cups water on a small saucepan to a boil. Once boiling, slow fire to a simmer and stir once. Cover and cook until water is fully absorbed and grains are soft around 15 minutes. Turn off fire, fluff grains with a fork and set aside to cool a bit.

Arrange one oven rack to highest position and preheat broiler. Line a baking sheet with foil, and grease with cooking spray.

Whisk well pepper, oil, rosemary, lemon juice and garlic. Rub onto chicken.

Place chicken on prepared pan, pop into the broiler and broil until juices run clear and no longer pin inside around 12 minutes.

Meanwhile, make the dressing by combining all ingredients in a blender. Blend until smooth.

Remove chicken from oven, cool slightly before cutting into strips, against the grain.

To assemble, place grains in a large salad bowl. Add in dressing and spinach, toss to mix well.

Add scallions and pear, mix gently and evenly divide into four plates. Top each salad with cheese and chicken.

Serve and enjoy.

Nutrition:

Calories 415

Fat 9g

Carbs 53g

Protein 30g

Fiber 7g

204. Grains and Fruits

Preparation Time: 10 Minutes

Cooking Time: 20 Minutes

Servings: 6

Ingredients:

¼ tsp salt

¾ cup bulgur

¾ cup quick cooking brown rice

1 8-oz low fat vanilla yogurt

1 cup raisins

1 Granny Smith apple

1 orange

1 Red delicious apple

3 cups water

Directions:

On high fire, place a large pot and bring water to a boil.

Add bulgur and rice. Lower fire to a simmer and cook for ten minutes while covered.

Turn off fire, set aside for 2 minutes while covered.

In baking sheet, transfer and evenly spread grains to cool.

Meanwhile, peel oranges and cut into sections. Chop and core apples.

Once grains are cool, transfer to a large serving bowl along with fruits.

Add yogurt and mix well to coat.

Serve and enjoy.

Nutrition:

Calories: 118 Cal

Fat: 1 g

Carbs: 24 g

Protein: 4 g

Fiber: 4 g

205. Cherries and Quinoa

Preparation Time: 5 Minutes

Cooking Time: 10 Minutes

Servings1

Ingredients:

1 tsp honey – optional

¼ tsp ground cinnamon

½ tsp vanilla extract

½ cup dried unsweetened cherries

½ cup dry quinoa

1 cup water

Directions:

Wash quinoa in a bowl, by rubbing vigorously between your hands. Discard water and repeat rinsing two more times.

On medium high fire, place a medium nonstick skillet.

Add cinnamon, vanilla extract, cherries and quinoa.

Bring to a boil and stir occasionally.

Once boiling, slow fire to a simmer, cover skillet and cook until all water is absorbed and quinoa is tender, around 15 minutes.

Turn off fire and let it stand covered for 10 minutes more.

Transfer to a serving bowl and if using honey, pour and mix.

Serve and enjoy.

Nutrition:

Calories: 386 Cal

Fat: 5.3 g

Carbs: 72.12 g

Protein: 13 g

Fiber: 7.7 g

206. Granola from Quinoa and Buckwheat

Preparation Time: 5 Minutes

Cooking Time: 45 Minutes

Servings: 6

Ingredients: ½ cup old fashioned oats

½ cup dried unsweetened cranberries

1 cup cooked quinoa 1 cup buckwheat groats

¼ tsp ground ginger ¼ tsp ground cinnamon

1 tsp vanilla extract 1 tbsp liquid coconut oil

3 tbsp honey

Directions:

Grease a baking sheet and preheat oven to 325oF.

In a large bowl, mix well oats, quinoa and buckwheat.

In a small bowl, stir well honey, coconut oil, vanilla, cinnamon, and ginger. Pour into bowl of oats and mix well. In an even layer, spread the mixture on baking sheet.

Pop into the oven and bake until grains begin to brown around 40 to 45 minutes.

Remove from oven and stir in cranberries.

Let it cool before serving or storing.

Nutrition:

Calories: 146 Cal Fat: 4 g Carbs: 29 g

Protein: 4 g Fiber: 3 g

207.   Trout 'n Cannellini Tartine

Preparation Time: 10 Minutes

Cooking Time: 0

Servings: 4

Ingredients: Dill sprigs – for garnish

4 large whole grain bread, toasted

1 tsp chopped fresh dill 2 tsp minced onion

1 stalk celery, finely chopped

½ 15-oz can cannellini beans

½ cup diced roasted red peppers

2 tbsp capers, rinsed and drained

¾ lb. smoked trout, flaked into bite-sized pieces

Pinch of sugar 1 tsp Dijon mustard

1 tbsp extra virgin olive oil

2 tbsp freshly squeezed lemon juice

Directions:

Mix sugar, mustard, olive oil and lemon juice in a big bowl. Add the rest of the ingredients except for toasted bread. Toss to mix well.

Evenly divide fish mixture on top of bread slices and garnish with dill sprigs. Serve and enjoy.

Nutrition:

Calories: 253 Cal Fat :9 g

Carbs 17 g Protein: 25 g Fiber: 4 g

208.   Chipotle Style Rice

Preparation Time: 10 Minutes

Cooking Time: 17 Minutes

Servings: 10

Ingredients:

1 can vegetable broth

1 cup water

2 tablespoons canola oil

3 tablespoons juice of lime juice

2 cups long grain brown rice, rinsed

Zest of 1 lime

½ cup cilantro, chopped

½ teaspoon salt

Directions:

Place everything in the pot and give a good stir, except for lime juice, lime zest, and cilantro.

Cover and bring to a boil. Boil for 5 minutes.

Lower fire to a simmer and cook until liquid is fully absorbed, around 10 to 15 minutes.

Mix in remaining ingredients and let it stand for another 5 minutes.

Fluff the rice before serving.

Nutrition:

Calories: 166 Cal Fat: 4g Carbs: 30g

Protein: 3 g Fiber: 1 g

209.   Rice & Currant Salad

Preparation Time: 10 Minutes

Cooking Time: 10 Minutes

Servings: 6

Ingredients:

1 cup brown basmati rice, uncooked

2 1/2 Tablespoons lemon juice

1 teaspoon grated orange zest

2 Tablespoons fresh orange juice

1/4 cup olive oil

1/2 teaspoon cinnamon

Salt and pepper to taste

4 chopped green onions

1/2 cup dried currants

3/4 cup shelled pistachios or almonds

1/4 cup chopped fresh parsley

Directions:

Place a nonstick pot on medium high fire and add rice. Toast rice until opaque and starts to smell, around 10 minutes.

Add 4 quarts of boiling water to pot and 2 tsp salt. Boil until tender, around 8 minutes uncovered.

Drain the rice and spread out on a lined cookie sheet to cool completely.

In a large salad bowl, whisk well the oil, juices and spices. Add salt and pepper to taste.

Add half of the green onions, half of parsley, currants, and nuts.

Toss with the cooled rice and let stand for at least 20 minutes.

If needed adjust seasoning with pepper and salt.

Garnish with remaining parsley and green onions.

Nutrition:

Calories: 365 Cal

Fat: 17 g

Carbs: 48 g

Protein: 8 g

Fiber: 5 g

210.   Quinoa Pilaf

Preparation Time: 10 Minutes

Cooking Time: 20 Minutes

Servings 10

Ingredients:

2 tablespoons onion, chopped

1 tablespoon garlic, minced

2 tablespoons chopped celery

2 cups quinoa, rinsed

2 cups chicken broth

¾ teaspoon garlic powder

¼ teaspoon paprika

Salt and pepper to taste

1 tablespoon parsley, chopped

Directions:

Mix broth and quinoa in a saucepan.

Bring to a boil and reduce to a simmer.

Cover and cook for 10 minutes.

Stir in onions, garlic, celery, garlic powder, paprika, salt, and pepper. Cover and continue cooking for another 5 minutes or until liquid is fully absorbed.

Once liquid is fully absorbed, turn off fire and let stand for 5 min.

Fluff with a fork, then stir in parsley.

Nutrition:

Calories: 132 Cal

Fat: 2 g

Carbs: 23 g

Protein: 5 g

Fiber :3 g

Sauces and Staples Recipes

211. Honey-Mustard-Sesame Sauce

Preparations Time: 10 Minutes

Cooking Time: 0

Servings: 1

Ingredients:

Dijon mustard – ½ cup

Raw honey or maple syrup – ½ cup

Garlic – 1 clove, minced

Toasted sesame oil - 1 tsp.

Directions:

In a bowl, add everything and whisk to mix.

Store in the refrigerator.

Nutrition:

Calories: 67 Cal

Fat: 1 g

Carb: 14 g

Protein: 1 g

212. Ginger-Teriyaki Sauce

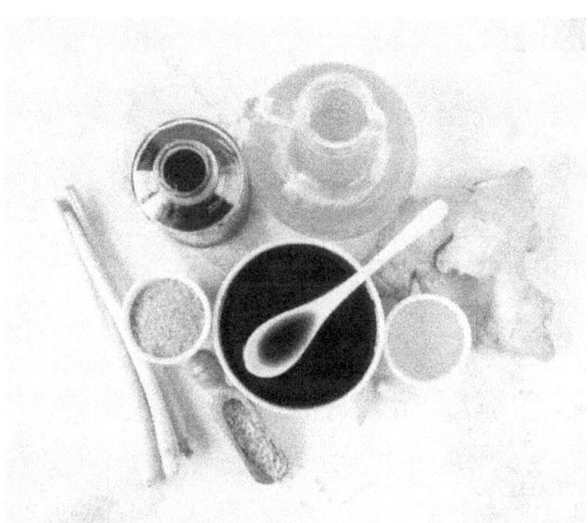

Preparation Time: 5 Minutes

Cooking Time: 0

Servings: 4

Ingredients Low sodium soy sauce – ¼ cup

No sugar added pineapple juice – ¼ cup

Raw honey – 2 Tbsps. Garlic powder – 1 tsp.

Grated fresh ginger - 1 Tbsp.

Arrowroot powder – 1 Tbsp.

Directions: Whisk everything in a bowl.

Store in the refrigerator.

Nutrition: Calories: 41 Cal Fat: 0 g

Carb: 10 g Protein: 1 g

213. Easy Garlicky Cherry Tomato Sauce

Preparation Time: 5 Minutes

Cooking Time: 25 Minutes

Servings: 4

Ingredients: ¼ cup extra virgin olive oil

¼ thinly sliced garlic cloves

2 pounds organic cherry tomatoes

½ teaspoon dried oregano

1 teaspoon coconut sugar

¼ cup chopped fresh basil 1 teaspoon salt

Directions:

Heat oil in a large saucepan over medium heat.

Sauté the garlic for a minute until fragrant.

Add in the cherry tomatoes and season with salt, oregano, coconut sugar, and fresh basil.

Allow to simmer for 25 minutes until the tomatoes are soft and becomes a thick sauce.

Place in containers and store in the fridge until ready to use.

Nutrition:

Calories: 198 Cal

Fat: 6 g

Carbs: 37 g Protein: 3 g

Fiber: 5 g

214. Avocado Cilantro Detox Dressing

Preparation Time: 5 Minutes

Cooking Time: 0

Servings 3

Ingredients:

5 tablespoons lemon juice, freshly squeezed

1 clove of garlic, chopped

1 avocado, pitted and flesh scooped out

1 bunch cilantro, chopped

¼ teaspoon salt

¼ cup water

Directions:

Place all ingredients in a food processor and pulse until well combined.

Pulse until creamy.

Place in a lidded container and store in the fridge until ready to use.

Use on salads and sandwiches.

Nutrition:

Calories 114 Cal

Fat: 10 g

Carbs: 8 g

Protein: 2 g Fiber: 5 g

215. Golden Turmeric Sauce

Preparation Time:10 Minutes

Cooking Time: 15 Minutes

Servings: 4

Ingredients: 2 tablespoons coconut oil

2-inch piece ginger, peeled and minced

2 cloves of garlic, minced

2 cups white sweet potato, cubed

2 tablespoons turmeric powder

½ teaspoon ginger powder

¼ teaspoon cinnamon powder

2 cups coconut milk 1 onion, chopped

Juice from 1 lemon, feshly squeezed

1 cup water 1 ½ teaspoon salt

Directions: Heat oil in a saucepan over medium flame. Sauté the onion, ginger, and garlic until fragrant. Add in the sweet potatoes, turmeric powder, ginger powder, and cinnamon powder. Pour in water and season with salt. Bring to a boil for 10 minutes. Once the potatoes are soft, place in a blender pulse until smooth. Return the mixture into the saucepan. Turn on the stove. Add in the coconut milk and lemon juice. Allow to simmer for 5 minutes. Store in lidded containers and put inside the fridge until ready to use.

Nutrition: Calories: 172 Cal Fat: 11 g

Carbs: 15 g Protein: 5 g Fiber: 3g

216. Creamy Turmeric Dressing

Preparation Time: 5 Minutes

Cooking Time: 0

Servings 6

Ingredients:

½ cup tahini

½ cup olive oil

2 tablespoons lemon juice

2 teaspoons honey

Salt to taste

a dash of black pepper

Directions:

Mix all ingredients in a bowl until the mixture becomes creamy and smooth.

Store in lidded containers.

Put in the fridge until ready to use.

Nutrition:

Calories 286

Fat 29g

Carbs 7g

Protein 4g

Fiber:2 g

217. Dijon Mustard Vinaigrette

Preparation Time: 5 Minutes

Cooking Time: 0

Servings: 6

Ingredients:

¾ cup olive oil

¼ cup apple cider vinegar

3 tablespoons Dijon mustard

2 shallots, quartered

1 garlic clove, chopped

A handful of parsley, chopped

Directions:

Place all ingredients in a food processor.

Pulse until smooth.

Place in containers and store in the fridge until ready to use.

Nutrition:

Calories: 252 Cal

Fat: 27 g

Carbs: 2 g

Protein: 0.6 g

Fiber: 0.7 g

218. Anti-Inflammatory Caesar Dressing

Preparation Time: 5 Minutes

Cooking Time: 0

Servings: 6

Ingredients:

½ cup cashew nuts, soaked in water then drained

1/3 cup fresh lemon juice

1 clove of garlic, minced

1 tablespoon Dijon mustard

1 tablespoon anchovy paste

2 tablespoon extra-virgin olive oil

½ cup plain Greek yogurt

Directions:

Place all ingredients in a food processor.

Pulse until a smooth paste is formed.

Place in containers and store in the fridge until ready to use.

Nutrition:

Calories: 96 Cal

Fat: 7 g

Carbs: 5 g

Protein: 4 g

Fiber: 0.5 g

219. Fresh Tomato Vinaigrette

Preparation Time: 5 Minutes

Cooking Time: 0

Servings 5

Ingredients:

1 fresh tomato, chopped

¾ cup olive oil

¼ cup apple cider vinegar

1 clove of garlic, chopped

½ teaspoon dried oregano

Salt and pepper to taste

Directions

Place all ingredients in a food processor.

Pulse until a smooth paste is formed.

Place in containers and store in the fridge until ready to use.

Nutrition:

Calories: 298 Cal

Fat: 32 g

Carbs: 2 g

Protein: 0.2 g

Fiber: 0.4 g

220. Ginger Sesame Sauce

Preparation Time: 5 Minutes

Cooking Time: 0

Servings: 6

Ingredients:

½ cup olive oil

¼ cup sesame oil

1/3 cup rice wine vinegar

1 tablespoon fresh ginger

1 tablespoon sesame seeds

Directions:

Place all ingredients in a food processor.

Pulse until a smooth paste is formed.

Place in containers and store in the fridge until ready to use.

Nutrition:

Calories: 250 Cal

Fat: 28 g

Carbs: 0.2 g

Protein: 0.3 g

Fiber: 0.1 g

221. Adobo Seasoning

Preparation Time: 10 Minutes

Cooking Time: 0

Servings: 40

Ingredients:

3 tablespoons garlic powder

1 teaspoon dried oregano, crushed

½ teaspoon ground cumin

2½ teaspoons salt

2 teaspoons freshly ground black pepper

Directions:

In a bowl, mix together all ingredients.

Store in an airtight jar.

Nutrition:

Calories: 3 Cal

Fat: 0 g

Carbs: 6 g

Fiber: 1 g

Protein: 1 g

222. Pumpkin Pie Spice

Preparation Time: 5 Minutes

Cooking Time: 0

Servings: 3

Ingredients:

1 teaspoon ground cinnamon

¼ teaspoon ground ginger

¼ teaspoon ground nutmeg

1/8 teaspoon ground cloves

Directions:

In a bowl, mix together all ingredients.

Store in an airtight jar.

Nutrition:

Calories: 6 Cal

Fat: 2g

Carbs: 4g

Fiber: 8g

Protein: 1g

223. Ginger-Garlic Paste

Preparation Time: 10 Minutes

Cooking Time: 0

Servings: 24

Ingredients:

4-ounce fresh ginger root, chopped

4-ounce garlic, chopped

1 tbsp olive oil

Directions:

In a food processor, add ginger and garlic and pulse till chopped finely.

While motor is running slowly, add oil and pulse till smooth.

Transfer the paste in an airtight jar and store in refrigerator.

Nutrition:

Calories: 24 Cal

Fat: 9g

Carbs: 6g

Fiber: 3g

Protein: 6g

224. Turmeric Paste

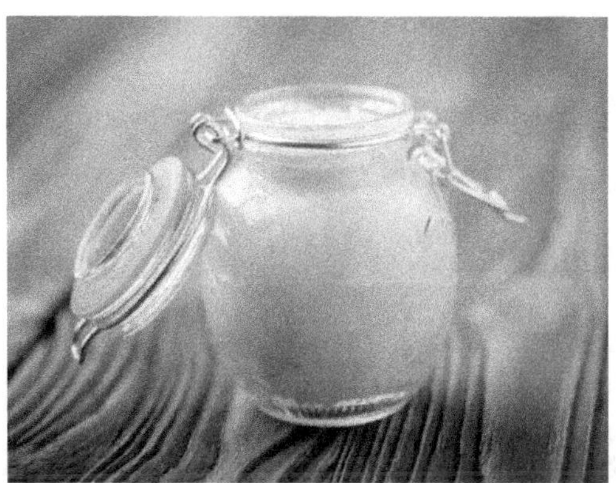

Preparation Time: 5 Minutes

Cooking Time: 0

Servings: 16

Ingredients:

1 cup raw honey

1 tablespoon coconut oil, softened

3 tablespoons ground turmeric

¼ teaspoon freshly ground black pepper

Directions:

In a sealable jar, add all ingredients and with a butter knife, mix well.

Refrigerate to store.

Nutrition:

Calories: 77 Cal

Fat: 1 g Carbs: 14 g

Fiber: 4 g

Protein: 2 g

225.   Garlicky Harissa

Preparation Time: 15 Minutes

Cooking Time: 4 Minutes

Servings: 16

Ingredients:

8 dried New Mexico chiles, stemmed and seeded

8 dried guajillochiles, stemmed and seeded

Boiling water, as required

½ teaspoon caraway seeds

¼ teaspoon cumin seeds

¼ teaspoon coriander seeds

1 teaspoon dried mint leaves

5 garlic cloves, chopped

3 tablespoons extra-virgin olive oil plus more, as needed

2 tablespoons fresh lemon juice

Salt, to taste

Directions:

In a bowl, add chiles and cover with boiling water.

Keep aside for about 20 minutes.

Meanwhile, heat a nonstick skillet on medium heat.

Add spice seeds and toast for about 4 minutes, swirling the skillet continuously.

In a grinder, add spice mixture and mint and pulse till powdered finely.

Drain the chiles completely.

In a food processor, add chiles, spice mixture and remaining ingredients and pulse till a smooth paste form.

Transfer the Harissa in a1-pint glass jar.

Add enough oil that will submerge the Harissa completely.

Nutrition:

Calories: 718 Cal

Fat: 0.9 g

Carbs: 11 g

Fiber: 5 g

Protein: 3 g

226.   Sweet Potato Sauce

Preparation Time: 15 Minutes

Cooking Time: 16 Minutes

Servings: 24

Ingredients:

2 tablespoons coconut oil

1 onion, chopped

2 minced garlic cloves

1- 2-inchpiece fresh ginger, minced

2 cups white sweet potato, peeled and cubed

1 cup bone broth

2 tablespoons ground turmeric

½ tablespoon ground ginger

¼ teaspoon ground cinnamon

Salt, to taste

1- 13½-ouncecan coconut milk

2 tablespoons fresh lemon juice

Directions:

In a pan, melt coconut oil on medium heat.

Add onion and sauté for about 5minutes.

Add garlic and ginger and sauté for about 1 minute.

Add sweet potato, broth and spices and bring to a boil.

Reduce the heat to low and simmer, covered for about 10 minutes.

Remove from heat and keep aside to cool for about 5 minutes.

In a blender, add sweet potato mixture and remaining ingredients and pulse till smooth.

Nutrition:

Calories: 76 Cal

Fat: 1 g

Carb: 11 g

Protein: 2 g

227. Tomato Sauce- Ketchup

Preparation Time: 15 Minutes

Cooking Time: 2 Hours 22 Minutes

Servings: 4-6

Ingredients:

1 tbsp olive oil

1 yellow onion, chopped

1- 1-inchpiece fresh ginger, minced

4 garlic cloves, minced

3 tablespoons tomato paste

1 teaspoon ground mustard

½ teaspoon cayenne pepper

½ teaspoon paprika

¼ teaspoon ground coriander

1/8 teaspoon ground cloves

2 bay leaves

1- 28-ouncecan diced tomatoes

¼ cup coconut crystals

½ cup coconut vinegar

Salt, to taste

Directions:

In a pan, heat oil on medium-high heat.

Add onion and sauté for about 5 minutes.

Add ginger and garlic and sauté for about 1 minute.

Stir in tomato paste and spices and sauté for about 1 minute.

Stir in remaining ingredients and reduce the heat to medium.

Simmer, stirring occasionally for about 15 minutes.

Remove from heat and keep aside to cool slightly.

In a blender, add tomato mixture and pulse till smooth.

Return the mixture into pan on low heat.

Simmer, stirring occasionally for about 2 hours.

Nutrition:

Calories: 97 Cal

Fat: 2 g

Carb: 24 g

Protein: 1 g

228. Scallion Sauce

Preparation Time: 15 Minutes

Cooking Time: 5 Minutes

Servings: 4-6

Ingredients:

2 cups scallions, chopped finely

1/3 cup fresh ginger, minced

1 teaspoon Aleppo pepper

Salt, to taste

¼ cup coconut oil

2 tablespoons extra-virgin olive oil

Directions:

In a large glass bowl, mix together all ingredients except both oils.

In a small pan, melt coconut oil for about 3-5 minutes.

Place the hot oil over scallion mixture evenly.

After 1-2 minutes, add olive oil and stir to combine well.

Nutrition:

Calories: 88 Cal

Fat: 0.7 g

Carb: 13 g

Protein: 3 g

229. Beet Sauce

Preparation Time: 15 Minutes

Cooking Time: 1 Hour

Servings: 6

Ingredients: 2 garlic cloves, chopped

2-pound beets, peeled and cubed

1 tablespoon coconut oil, melted

2 tablespoons fresh lemon juice

1 tablespoon apple cider vinegar

¼ cup water Salt, to taste

1/3 cup extra-virgin olive oil

Directions:

Preheat the oven to 400 degrees F.

Coat the beet cubes with coconut oil evenly.

Place the beet cubes in a baking dish.

Bake for about 1 hour, stirring after every 20 minutes.

Remove from oven and keep aside to cool for about 10 minutes.

In a food processor, add beets and remaining ingredients except olive oil and pulse till well combined.

While motor is running slowly, add oil pulsing continuously till smooth.

Nutrition: Calories: 57 Cal Fat: 19 g

Carb:27 g Protein: 7 g

230. Eggplant Sauce- Baba Ghanoush

Preparation Time: 15 Minutes

Cooking Time: 35 Minutes

Servings: 8

Ingredients: 2 large eggplants

2 garlic cloves, chopped 2 tablespoons tahini

2 tablespoons fresh lemon juice

3 teaspoons extra-virgin olive oil

1 teaspoon ground cumin

Salt and freshly ground black pepper, to taste

Olive oil, for drizzling

Chopped fresh parsley leaves, for garnishing

Directions:

Preheat the oven to 400 degrees F. Grease a baking dish. Place the eggplants in prepared baking dish.

Bake for about 35 minutes.

Remove from oven and immediately, place in bowl of cold water to cool slightly.

Peel off the skin of eggplants.

In a food processor, add eggplants and remaining ingredients except olive oil and parsley and pulse till smooth.

Refrigerate to chill before.

While, drizzle with olive oil and garnish with parsley.

Vegetarian and Vegan Recipes

231. Nutty and Fruity Garden Salad

Preparation time: 10 minutes

Cooking time: 0 minutes

Servings: 2

Ingredients: 6 cups baby spinach

½ cup chopped walnuts, toasted

1 ripe red pear, sliced

1 ripe persimmon, sliced

1 teaspoon garlic minced   1 shallot, minced

1 tablespoon extra-virgin olive oil

2 tablespoons fresh lemon juice

1 teaspoon whole grain mustard

Directions:

Mix well garlic, shallot, oil, lemon juice and mustard in a large salad bowl.

Add spinach, pear and persimmon. Toss to coat well.

To serve, garnish with chopped pecans.

Nutrition:

Calories 332 Fat 21g Carbs 37g

Protein 7g Fiber 9g

232. Creamy Cauliflower-Broccoli Soup

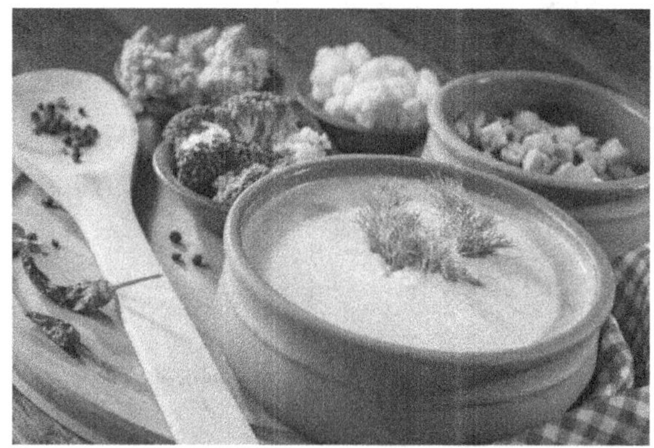

Preparation time: 15 minutes

Cooking time: 15 minutes

Servings: 6

Ingredients:

Pepper and salt to taste

4 cups chicken broth

1 teaspoon dried basil

1 teaspoon dried oregano

½ cup onion, roughly chopped

2 cups carrots, cubed

3 cups cauliflower florets

2 cups broccoli florets

Directrions:

In a large soup pot, bring to a boil chicken broth, basil, oregano and onions. Once boiling, lower fire to a simmer.

Meanwhile, dice cauliflower and broccoli florets. And add to pot. Add carrots, cover and simmer for 10 minutes. Season with pepper and salt to taste.

Turn off fire and allow soup to cool.

Place veggies into a blender while ensuring that liquid is reserved. Puree veggies along with 1 cup of reserved liquid. If you want a thick soup, then 1 cup liquid is enough. If you desire a less thick soup, add more reserved liquid until desired consistency is reached.

Return pureed soup to empty pot and simmer until heated through. Adjust seasoning if needed before serving.

Nutrition:

Calories 39

Fat 0.3g

Carbs 8g

Protein 2g

Fiber 3g

233. Nutty and Fruity Amaranth Porridge

Preparation time: 10 minutes

Cooking time: 30 minutes

Servings: 2

Ingredients:

1 medium pear, chopped

½ cup blueberries

1 tsp cinnamon

1 tbsp raw honey

¼ cup pumpkin seeds

2 cups filtered water

2/3 cups whole-grain amaranth

Directions:

In a nonstick pan with cover, boil water and amaranth. Slow fire to a simmer and continue cooking until liquid is absorbed completely, around 25-30 minutes.

Turn off fire.

Mix in cinnamon, honey and pumpkin seeds. Mix well.

Pour equally into two bowls.

Garnish with pear and blueberries.

Serve and enjoy.

Nutrition: Calories 416 Fat 12g

Carbs 68g Protein 14g Fiber 7g

234.   Korean Barbecue Tofu

Preparation time: 10 minutes

Cooking time: 15 minutes

Servings: 3

Ingredients: 1 tbsp olive oil

2 tsp onion powder

4 garlic cloves, minced   2 tsp dry mustard

3 tbsp brown sugar   ½ cup soy sauce

1 ½ lbs. firm tofu, sliced to ¼-inch cubes

Directions

In a re-sealable bag, mix all ingredients except for tofu and oil. Mix well until sugar is dissolved.

Add sliced tofu and slowly turn bag to mmix. Seal bag and place flatly inside the ref for an hour.

After an hour, turn bag to the other side and marinate for another hour.

To cook, in a nonstick fry pan, heat oil on medium high fire. Add tofu and stir fry until sides are browned.

Serve and enjoy.

Nutrition: Calories 437

Fat 25g Carbs 23g

Protein 40g

Fiber 6g

235.   Fruit Bowl with Yogurt Topping

Preparation time: 15 minutes

Cooking time: 0 minutes

Servings: 6

Ingredients: ¼ cup golden brown sugar

2/3 cup minced fresh ginger

1 16-oz Greek yogurt

¼ tsp ground cinnamon   2 tbsp honey

½ cup dried cranberries

3 navel oranges   2 large tangerines

1 pink grapefruit, peeled

Directions:

Into sections, break tangerines and grapefruit.

Slice tangerine sections in half and grapefruit sections into thirds. Place all sliced fruits and its juices in a large bowl.

Peel oranges, remove pith, slice into ¼-inch thick rounds and then cut into quarters. Transfer to bowl of fruit along with juices. In bowl, add cinnamon, honey and ¼ cup of cranberries. Place in the ref for an hour. In a medium bowl mix ginger and yogurt. Place on top of fruit bowl, drizzle with remaining cranberries and brown sugar.

Serve and enjoy.

Nutrition: Calories 171 Fat 1g

Carbs 35g Protein 9g Fiber 3g

236. Mushroom, Spinach and Turmeric Frittata

Preparation time: 10 minutes

Cooking time: 40 minutes

Servings: 6

Ingredients:

½ tsp pepper

½ tsp salt

1 tsp turmeric

5-oz firm tofu

4 large eggs

6 large egg whites

¼ cup water

1 lb. fresh spinach

6 cloves freshly chopped garlic

1 large onion, chopped

1 lb. button mushrooms, sliced

Directions:

Grease a 10-inch nonstick and oven proof skillet and preheat oven to 350oF.

Place skillet on medium high fire and add mushrooms. Cook until golden brown.

Add onions, cook for 3 minutes or until onions are tender.

Add garlic, sauté for 30 seconds.

Add water and spinach, cook while covered until spinach is wilted, around 2 minutes.

Remove lid and continue cooking until water is fully evaporated.

 In a blender, puree pepper, salt, turmeric, tofu, eggs and egg whites until smooth. Pour into skillet once liquid is fully evaporated.

Pop skillet into oven and bake until the center is set around 25-30 minutes.

Remove skillet from oven and let it stand for ten minutes before inverting and transferring to a serving plate.

Cut into 6 equal wedges, serve and enjoy.

Nutrition:

Calories 358

Fat 6g

Carbs 65g

Protein 21g

Fiber 12g

237.   Roasted Root Vegetables

Preparation time: 10 minutes

Cooking time: 1 hour and 30 minutes

Servings: 6

Ingredients:

2 tbsp olive oil

1 head garlic, cloves separated and peeled

1 large turnip, peeled and cut into ½-inch pieces

1 medium sized red onion, cut into ½-inch pieces

1 ½ lbs. beets, trimmed but not peeled, scrubbed and cut into ½-inch pieces

1 ½ lbs. Yukon gold potatoes, unpeeled, cut into ½-inch pieces

2 ½ lbs. butternut squash, peeled, seeded, cut into ½-inch pieces

Directions:

Grease 2 rimmed and large baking sheets. Preheat oven to 425oF.

In a large bowl, mix all ingredients thoroughly.

Into the two baking sheets, evenly divide the root vegetables, spread in one layer.

Season generously with pepper and salt.

Pop into the oven and roast for 1 hour and 15 minute or until golden brown and tender.

Remove from oven and let it cool for at least 15 minutes before serving.

Nutrition:

Calories 278 Fat 5g

Carbs 57g Protein 6g Fiber 10g

238.   Tropical Fruit Parfait

Preparation time: 10 minutes

Cooking time: 10 minutes

Servings: 1

Ingredients:

1 tbsp toasted sliced almonds

¼ cup plain soy yogurt

½ cup of fruit combination cut into ½-inch cubes (pineapple, mango and kiwi)

Instructions:

Prepare fresh fruit by peeling and slicing into ½-inch cubes.

Place cubed fruit in a bowl and top with a dollop of soy yogurt.

Garnish with sliced almonds and if desired, refrigerate for an hour before serving.

Nutrition:

Calories 119 Fat 2g

Carbs 25g Protein 2g Fiber 1g

239. Cinnamon Chips with Avocado-Strawberry Salsa

Preparation time: 10 minutes

Cooking time: 10 minutes

Servings: 6

Ingredients:

3/8 tsp salt

2 tsp fresh lime juice

1 tsp minced seeded jalapeno pepper

2 tbsp minced fresh cilantro

1 cup finely chopped strawberries

1 ½ cups finely chopped, peeled and ripe avocado

½ tsp ground cinnamon

2 tsp sugar

6 6-inch brown rice tortillas

2 tsp olive oil

Directions:

Preheat oven to 350oF.

Prepare the cinnamon chips by brushing olive oil all over the brown rice tortilla.

In a small bowl, mix together cinnamon and sugar.

Sprinkle cinnamon-sugar mixture evenly all over each of the brown rice tortilla.

Cut up each tortilla into 12 wedges, evenly and place on a baking sheet. If needed you can bake tortilla in two batches.

Pop the tortillas into the oven and bake until crisped, around 10 minutes. Remove from oven and keep warm.

Meanwhile, prepare salsa by mixing the remaining ingredients in a medium bowl. Stir to mix well.

To enjoy, dip crisped tortillas into bowl of salsa and eat or, you can spread the fruity salsa all over one tortilla chip and enjoy.

Nutrition:

Calories 213

Fat 11g

Carbs 25g

Protein 5g

Fiber 7g

240. Stir Fried Brussels Sprouts and Carrots

Preparation time: 10 minutes

Cooking time: 15 minutes

Servings: 6

Ingredients:

1 tbsp cider vinegar

1/3 cup water

1 lb. Brussels sprouts, halved lengthwise

1 lb. carrots cut diagonally into ½-inch thick lengths

3 tbsp olive oil, divided

2 tbsp chopped shallot

½ tsp pepper

¾ tsp salt

Directions:

On medium high fire, place a nonstick medium fry pan and heat 2 tbsp oil.

Ass shallots and cook until softened, around one to two minutes while occasionally stirring.

Add pepper salt, Brussels sprouts and carrots. Stir fry until vegetables starts to brown on the edges, around 3 to 4 minutes.

Add water, cook and cover.

After 5 to 8 minutes, or when veggies are already soft, add remaining butter.

If needed season with more pepper and salt to taste.

Turn off fire, transfer to a platter, serve and enjoy.

Nutrition:

Calories 98 Fat 4g Carbs 14g

Protein 3 Fiber 5g

241. Curried Veggies and Poached Eggs

Preparation time: 10 minutes

Cooking time: 50 minutes

Servings: 4

Ingredients: 4 large eggs

½ tsp white vinegar

1/8 tsp crushed red pepper – optional

1 cup water

1 14-oz can chickpeas, drained

2 medium zucchinis, diced

½ lb. sliced button mushrooms

1 tbsp yellow curry powder

2 cloves garlic, minced

1 large onion, chopped

2 tsp extra virgin olive oil

Directions:

On medium high fire, place a large saucepan and heat oil.

Sauté onions until tender around four to five minutes.

Add garlic and continue sautéing for another half minute.

Add curry powder, stir and cook until fragrant around one to two minutes.

Add mushrooms, mix, cover and cook for 5 to 8 minutes or until mushrooms are tender and have released their liquid.

Add red pepper if using, water, chickpeas and zucchini. Mix well to combine and bring to a boil.

Once boiling, reduce fire to a simmer, cover and cook until zucchini is tender around 15 to 20 minutes of simmering.

Meanwhile, in a small pot filled with 3-inches deep of water, bring to a boil on high fire.

Once boiling, reduce fire to a simmer and add vinegar.

Slowly add one egg, slipping it gently into the water. Allow to simmer until egg is cooked, around 3 to 5 minutes.

Remove egg with a slotted spoon and transfer to a plate, one plate one egg.

Repeat the process with remaining eggs.

Once the veggies are done cooking, divide evenly into 4 servings and place one serving per plate of egg.

Serve and enjoy.

Nutrition: Calories 254 Fat 9g Carbs 30g

Protein 16g Fiber 9g

242.   Braised Kale

Preparation Time: 10minutes

Cooking Time: 15 minutes

Servings 3

Ingredients: 2 to 3 tbsp water

1 tbsp coconut oil ½ sliced red pepper

2 stalk celery (sliced to ¼-inch thick)

5 cups of chopped kale

Directions:

Heat a pan over medium heat. Add coconut oil and sauté the celery for at least five minutes. Add the kale and red pepper.

Add a tablespoon of water.

Let the vegetables wilt for a few minutes. Add a tablespoon of water if the kale starts to stick to the pan. Serve warm.

Nutrition: Calories 61 Fat 5g

Carbs 3g Protein 1g

Fiber 1g,

243.   Braised Leeks, Cauliflower and Artichoke Hearts

Preparation Time: 10 minutes

Cooking Time: 10 minutes

Servings 4

Ingredients:

2 tbsp coconut oil

2 garlic cloves, chopped

1 ½ cup artichoke hearts

1 ½ cups chopped leeks

1 ½ cups cauliflower flowerets

Directions:

Heat oil in a skillet over medium high heat.

Add the garlic and sauté for one minute. Add the vegetables and stir constantly until the vegetables are cooked.

Serve with roasted chicken, fish or pork.

Nutrition:

Calories 111

Fat 7g

Carbs 12g

Protein 3g

Fiber 4g

244.   Celery Root Hash Browns

Preparation Time: 10 minutes

Cooking Time: 10 minutes

Servings 4

Ingredients:

4 tbsp coconut oil

½ tsp sea salt

2 to 3 medium celery roots

Directions:

Scrub the celery root clean and peel it using a vegetable peeler.

Grate the celery root in a food processor or a manual grater.

In a skillet, add oil and heat it over medium heat.

Place the grated celery root on the skillet and sprinkle with salt.

Let it cook for 10 minutes on each side or until the grated celery turns brown.

Serve warm.

Nutrition:

Calories 160

Fat 14g Fat 3g

Carbs 10g

Protein 1.5g Fiber 3g

245. Zucchini Pasta with Avocado Sauce

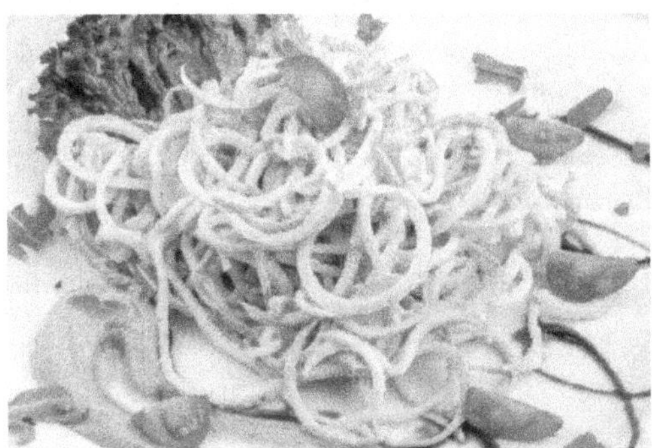

Preparations Time: 10 minutes

Cooking Time: 10 minutes

Servings 1

Ingredients: A squeeze of lemon juice

Salt and pepper to taste 1 tbsp coconut milk

½ ripe avocado 2 tbsp olive oil

1 medium zucchini cut into noodles

Directions:

Heat the oil in a skillet over medium heat and add the zucchini noodles. Sauté for three minutes or until the noodles have softened.

While the zucchini is cooking, mash the avocado together with the coconut milk, lemon juice and salt and pepper. Add the sauce to the zucchini noodles and sauté. Serve warm.

Nutrition: Calories 471 Fat 43g

Carbs 23g Protein 6g Fiber 9g

Blueberry Chia Pudding

Preparations Time: 10 minutes

Cooking Time: 10 minutes

Servings 2

Ingredients:

½ cup chia seeds

½ of frozen banana

5 dates (soaked in water)

2/3 cup almond milk

2 cups frozen blueberries

Directions:

Combine the milk, blueberries, dates and bananas in a blender. Process until the mixture becomes smooth.

Transfer the blueberry to a bowl and add the chia seeds.

Refrigerate for 30 minutes or overnight if necessary, until the chia seeds forms mucilage.

Serve with your favorite fruit or nut toppings.

Nutrition:

Calories 343

Fat 13g

Carbs 55g

Protein 9g

Fiber 16g,

Collard Green Wrap

Preparation Time: 10 minutes

Cooking Time: 0 minutes

Servings 4

Ingredients:

½ block feta, cut into 4 (1-inch thick) strips (4-oz)

½ cup purple onion, diced

½ medium red bell pepper, julienned

1 medium cucumber, julienned

4 large cherry tomatoes, halved

4 large collard green leaves, washed

8 whole kalamata olives, halved

Sauce Ingredients:

1 cup low-fat plain Greek yogurt

1 tablespoon white vinegar

1 teaspoon garlic powder

2 tablespoons minced fresh dill

2 tablespoons olive oil

2.5-ounces cucumber, seeded and grated (¼-whole)

Salt and pepper to taste

Directions:

Make the sauce first: make sure to squeeze out all the excess liquid from the cucumber after grating. In a small bowl, mix all sauce ingredients thoroughly and refrigerate.

Prepare and slice all wrap ingredients.

On a flat surface, spread one collard green leaf. Spread 2 tablespoons of Tzatziki sauce on middle of the leaf.

Layer ¼ of each of the tomatoes, feta, olives, onion, pepper, and cucumber. Place them on the center of the leaf, like piling them high instead of spreading them.

Fold the leaf like you would a burrito. Repeat process for remaining ingredients.

Serve and enjoy.

Nutrition:

Calories 463

Fat 31g

Carbs 31g

Protein 20g

Fiber 7g

246. Zucchini Garlic Fries

Preparation Time: 10 minutes

Cooking Time: 20 minutes

Servings 6

Ingredients:

¼ teaspoon garlic powder

½ cup almond flour

2 large egg whites, beaten

3 medium zucchinis, sliced into fry sticks

Salt and pepper to taste

Directions:

Preheat oven to 400oF.

Mix all ingredients in a bowl until the zucchini fries are well coated.

Place fries on cookie sheet and spread evenly.

Put in oven and cook for 20 minutes.

Halfway through cooking time, stir fries.

Nutrition:

Calories 11

Fat 0.1g,

Carbs 1g

Protein1.5 g

Fiber 0.5g

247. Mashed Cauliflower

Preparation Time: 10 minutes

Cooking Time: 10 minutes

Servings 3

Ingredients:

1 cauliflower head

1 tablespoon olive oil

½ tsp salt

¼ tsp dill

Pepper to taste

2 tbsp low fat milk

Directions:

Bring a small pot of water to a boil.

Chop cauliflower in florets.

Add florets to boiling water and boil uncovered for 5 minutes. Turn off fire and let it sit for 5 minutes more.

In a blender, add all ingredients except for cauliflower and blend to mix well.

Drain cauliflower well and add into blender. Puree until smooth and creamy.

Serve and enjoy.

Nutrition: Calories 78

Fat 5g Carbs 6g

Protein 2g Fiber 2g

248. Stir-Fried Eggplant

Preparation Time: 10 minutes

Cooking Time: 10 minutes

Servings 2

Ingredients: 1 tablespoon coconut oil

2 eggplants, sliced into 3-inch in length

4 cloves of garlic, minced

1 onion, chopped 1 teaspoon ginger, grated

1 teaspoon lemon juice, freshly squeezed

½ tsp salt

½ tsp pepper

Directions:

Heat oil in a nonstick saucepan.

Pan-fry the eggplants for 2 minutes on all sides.

Add the garlic and onions until fragrant, around 3 minutes.

Stir in the ginger, salt, pepper, and lemon juice.

Add a ½ cup of water and bring to a simmer. Cook until eggplant is tender.

Nutrition:

Calories 232

Fat 8g Carbs 41g

Protein 7g Fiber 18g

249. Sautéed Garlic Mushrooms

Preparation Time: 10 minutes

Cooking Time: 10 minutes

Servings 4

Ingredients:

1 tablespoon olive oil

3 cloves of garlic, minced

16 ounces fresh brown mushrooms, sliced

7 ounces fresh shiitake mushrooms, sliced

½ tsp salt

½ tsp pepper or more to taste

Directions:

Place a nonstick saucepan on medium high fire and heat pan for a minute.

Add oil and heat for 2 minutes.

Stir in garlic and sauté for a minute.

Add remaining ingredients and stir fry until soft and tender, around 5 minutes.

Turn off fire, let mushrooms rest while pan is covered for 5 minutes.

Serve and enjoy.

Nutrition:

Calories 95 Fat 4g Carbs 14g Protein 3g,

Fiber 4g

250. Stir Fried Asparagus and Bell Pepper

Preparation Time: 10 minutes

Cooking Time: 10 minutes

Servings 6

Ingredients:

1 tablespoon olive oil

4 cloves of garlic, minced

1-pound fresh asparagus spears, trimmed

2 large red bell peppers, seeded and julienned

½ teaspoon thyme

5 tablespoons water

½ tsp salt

½ tsp pepper or more to taste

Directions:

Place a nonstick saucepan on high fire and heat pan for a minute.

Add oil and heat for 2 minutes.

Stir in garlic and sauté for a minute.

Add remaining ingredients and stir fry until soft and tender, around 6 minutes.

Turn off fire, let veggies rest while pan is covered for 5 minutes.

Nutrition:

Calories 45

Fat 2g

Carbs 5g, Net

Protein 2g

Fiber 2g

Dessert Recipes

251.   A Skillet Full of Granola

Preparation Time: 7 Minutes

Cooking Time: 12 Minutes

Servings: 3

Ingredients   6 pieces of pitted Mejdool dates

¼ cup of boiling water

1 tablespoon of coconut oil (melted)

1 tablespoon of cinnamon

¼ teaspoon of sea salt 2 cups of rolled oats

1 cup of raw nuts

Directions:

Take a food processor and add water, dates, cinnamon, oil, salt and puree the whole mixture until smooth Transfer it to a large sized bowl and stir in your oats, seeds and nuts Take a 12 inch skillet and place it over medium heat Add the mixture and cook it for about 12 minutes, making sure to keep stirring it regularly   Let it cool and serve!

Nutrition:

Calories: 132 Cal Fat: 6 g

Carbs: 18 g Protein: 2.8 g

252.   Feisty Chia and Oatmeal Cookies

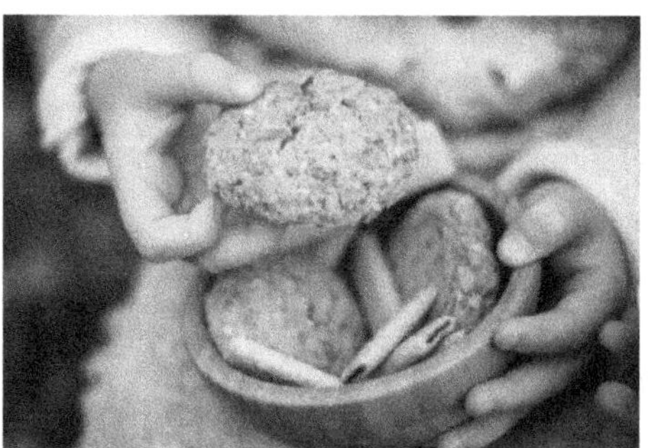

Preparation Time: 15 Minutes

Cooking Time: 10 Minutes

Servings: 4

Ingredients:

2 cups of rolled oatmeal

1 cup of brown sugar

2/3 cup of whole wheat flour

2 tablespoon of chia seeds

1 teaspoon of cinnamon, ground

1 teaspoon of baking soda

½ a teaspoon of baking powder

½ a teaspoon of salt

2/3 cup of applesauce

3 tablespoon of coconut oil

1 cup of dried cranberries

½ a cup of chocolate chips

¼ cup of unsweetened coconut, shredded

Directions:

Pre-heat your oven to 350-degree Fahrenheit

Take a bowl and add oats, flour, sugar, chia seeds, baking soda, cinnamon, baking powder and salt

Line up a baking sheet with parchment paper

Mix well

Stir in your applesauce alongside coconut oil into the oat mix and keep mixing until you have a even dough

Fold in chocolate chips (if using), cranberries and coconut

Spoon up the dough into your baking sheet

Bake for 10-15 minutes and enjoy!

Nutrition:

Calories: 262 Cal

Fats: 8 g

Carbs:47 g

Protein:3.4 g

253. Traditional Orange (Vegan) Cake

Preparation Time: 15 Minutes

Cooking Time: 30 Minutes

Servings: 4

Ingredients   1 large sized orange, peeled

1 and a ½ cups of all-purpose flour

1 cup of white sugar   ½ a cup of vegetable oil

1 and a ½ teaspoon of baking soda

¼ teaspoon of salt

Directions:

Pre-heat your oven to 375 degree Fahrenheit

Take an 8x8 inch baking pan and grease it up well

Take a blender and blend in orange, making sure to get at least 1 cup of orange juice

Take a bowl and whisk in orange juice, vegetable oil, sugar, baking soda, and salt

Mix well and pour the prepared batter into your pan

Bake for about 30 minutes until a toothpick comes out clean from the center

Enjoy!

Nutrition: Calories: 157 Cal

Fats: 7 g Carbs:22 g Protein:1.3 g

254. Ravishing Choco-Nut Banana Bites

Preparation Time: 10 Minutes

Cooking Time: 0

Servings: 4

Ingredients:

4 teaspoons of cocoa powder

4 teaspoons of toasted unsweetened coconut

2 sliced of small bananas

Directions:

Take two individual plates and place the cocoa and coconut on those plates (individually)

Roll up the banana slices in the cocoa first and shake off any excess

Then dip them in the coconut

Serve!

Nutrition:

Protein: 1 g

Carbs: 13 g

Fats: 1 g

Calories: 60 Cal

255. Very Cool And "Offbeat" Melon Soup

Preparation Time: 15 Minutes

Cooking Time: 0

Servings: 4

Ingredients

4 cups of casaba melon, cubed and seeded

¾ cup of coconut milk

Juice of 2 lime

1 tablespoon ginger, grated

1 pinch of salt

Directions:

Add the coconut milk, casaba melon, lime juice, salt and ginger to your food processor

Process it for about 1-2 minutes until the mixture has a soup like texture

Enjoy!

Nutrition:

Calories: 134 Cal

Fats: 9 g

Carbs:13 g

Protein:2 g

256. Fantastic Almond "Vegan" Butter Balls

Preparation Time: 10 Minutes

Cooking Time: 0

Servings: 4

Ingredients

12 dates, pitted and diced

1/3 cup of unsweetened shredded coconut

2 and a ½ tablespoon of almond butter

Directions:

Take a bowl and add dates, almond butter and coconut

Mix well

Use the mixture to form small balls

Store them in your fridge and chill them

Enjoy!

Nutrition:

Calories: 62 Cal

Fats: 3 g

Carbs:8 g

Protein:1 g

257. Fancy Coconut Date Bars For A Lovely Evening

Preparation Time: 10 Minutes

Cooking Time: 30 Minutes

Servings: 4

Ingredients:

1/3 cup of slivered almonds

½ a cup coconut, flaked

10 dates, pitted

¼ cup of cashews

1 teaspoon of coconut oil

Directions:

Take a food processor and ad the almonds, blend them

Add dates and pulse until mixed well

Add coconut oil and cashews until the mix is thick and sticks together

Transfer the mixture to a wax paper and form nice squares

Fold up the sides of the waxed-on top

Chill for at least 30 minutes and serve

Enjoy!

Nutrition: Calories: 154 Cal

Fats: 0 g Carbs: 39 g

Protein: 0.1 g

258. Vegan Coconut Whipped Cream

Preparation Time: 8 Hours 10 Minutes

Cook Time: 0

Servings: 6

Ingredients: 2 tablespoons of white sugar

1 can of unsweetened coconut milk

1 teaspoon of pure vanilla extract

Directions:

Place the can of coconut in your fridge and allow it to chill for 8 hours

Make sure to chill a metal bowl and beats in your fridge for about 1 hour prior to preparing the whip

Open up your coconut milk can and scoop out the coconut cream solids into your metal bowl Keep the liquids for later use

Beat the cream using a mixer on medium speed

Set the speed on HIGH and beat for 7-8 minutes until stiff peaks form

Add sugar, vanilla extract to the coconut cream and beat for 1 minute more Give it a taste and add more sugar if needed

Enjoy with cakes of muffins!

Nutrition:

Calories: 11 Cal Fats: 0 g

Carbs: 2.4 g Protein: 0 g

259. Thar She' Salts Peanut Butter Cookies

Preparation Time: 15 Minutes

Cooking Time: 0

Servings: 9

Ingredients

1 cup of raw almonds

½ a cup of peanut butter (creamy and unsalted)

1 cup of pitted Mejdool dates

1 and a ¼ teaspoon of vanilla extract

Sea salt as needed

Directions:

Take a food processor and add almonds, peanut butter, vanilla, dates and blend the whole mixture until a dough like texture comes (should take a few minutes)

Add some more peanut butter if you want a stickier dough

Form balls using the dough and press down using fork to create a criss cross pattern

Sprinkle salt generously

Serve immediately or allow it to chill for crunchiness

Nutrition:

Calories: 350 Cal Fat: 17 g Carbs: 27 g

Protein: 18 g

260. A Snowy "Frozen" Salad Bowl

Preparation Time: 75 Minutes

Cooking Time: 0

Servings: 3

Ingredients: ½ a cup of white sugar

2 cups of water

1 can of 20-ounce frozen orange juice concentrate (thawed)

1 can of 20-ounce frozen lemonade concentrated (thawed)

4 bananas, sliced

1 can of crushed pineapple (with juice)

1 pack of strawberries (thawed)

Directions:

Take a bowl and add water and sugar

Dissolve the sugar and add orange juice, bananas, lemonade, crushed pineapples (alongside the juice), strawberries and give it a nice mix

Pour the mixture into a 9x13 inch glass pan and allow it to chill

Once ready to serve, let it sit for about 5 minutes at room temp and cut them out

Nutrition: Calories: 350 Cal

Fats: 0.5 g Carbs: 89 g

Protein: 2.5 g

261. Age Old Poached Pears

Preparation Time: 3 Minutes

Cooking Time: 17 Minutes

Servings: 4

Ingredients: 3 and a ½ cups of water

3 semi ripe pears (preferably Barlett pears)

3 cups of granulated sugar

Rind of 1 lemon Juice of 1 lemon

1 teaspoon of vanilla extract

2 cinnamon sticks

2 pieces of whole cloves 1 whole star anise

Directions:

Peel your pears and keep them on the side

Take a pot and add vanilla extract, water, lemon juice, sugar, lemon rind, star anise, cinnamon sticks and cloves

Place it over medium heat and keep Cook until the sugar dissolves

Add your peas and lower down the heat to low Allow it to simmer for 15-20 minutes

Once the pears are soft, transfer to a Tupperware with Cook liquid Allow it to cool

Serve and enjoy!

Nutrition:

Calories: 740 Cal Fat: 4 g Carbs: 180 g

Protein: 4 g

262. A Pineapple "Sherbet" If You Please

Preparation Time: 20 Minutes

Cooking Time: 0

Servings: 4

Ingredients

1 can of 8-ounce pineapple chunks

1/3 cup of orange marmalade

¼ teaspoon of ground ginger

¼ teaspoon of vanilla extract

1 can of 11-ounce orange sections

2 cups of pineapple, lemon or lime sherbet

Directions:

Drain the pineapple, making sure to reserve the juice. Take a medium sized bowl and add pineapple juice, ginger, vanilla and marmalade to the bowl. Add pineapple chunks, drained mandarin oranges as well. Toss well and coat everything

Free them for 15 minutes and allow them to chill

Spoon the sherbet into 4 chilled stemmed sherbet dishes. Top each of them with fruit mixture. Enjoy!

Nutrition: Calories: 267 Cal Fat: 1 g

Carbs: 65 g Protein: 2 g

263. Very Rough and Tough Fried Apple

Preparation Time: 10 Minutes

Cooking Time: 10 Minute

Servings: 4

Ingredients

½ a cup of vegan butter

½ a cup of white sugar

2 tablespoon of ground cinnamon

4 Granny Smith Apples, peeled, sliced and cored

Directions:

Take a large sized skillet and place it over medium hat

Add the vegan butter and allow it to melt

Stir in cinnamon and sugar into the melted butter

Add the cut up apples and cook them nicely for about 5-8 minutes until they break down

Enjoy!

Nutrition:

Calories: 369 Cal

Fat: 23 g

Carbs: 44 g

Protein: 1 g

264. Mind Blowing Tofu "Mocha" Bars

Preparation Time: 5 Minutes

Cooking Time: 10 Minutes

Servings: 3

Ingredients: 2 tablespoon of safflower oil

12 ounces of silken tofu (make sure to not drain it)

Just a pinch of salt 2 and a 1/3 cups of sugar

1 cup of cocoa powder

1/3 cup of instant coffee powder (decaf)

1 teaspoon of vanilla extract

1 cup of whole wheat flour

Directions:

Pre-heat your oven to 325-degree Fahrenheit. Take an electric mixer and blend tofu until a creamy texture is obtained. Add salt, oil, cocoa, sugar coffee and vanilla and blend it again. Once the sugar has dissolved, remove the mixture from your blender and whisk in flour. Pour the batter into a greased up 9x13 inch baking pan. Bake for about 25-30 minutes until the cake starts to pull away from the sides of the pan. The bar should give you a glossy finish, take them out and allow it to cool. Cut them using a clean (wet) knife and serve!

Nutrition: Calories: 117 Fats: 2g

Carbs: 24g Protein: 2.4g

265. Tapioca Strawberry Mix

Preparation Time: 15 Minutes

Cooking Time: 0

Servings: 4

Ingredients

½ a cup of fresh strawberries, halved and hulled

1 and a ½ cup of water

¼ cup of quick-Cook tapioca

Directions:

Take your blender and add the berries alongside water

Process for a few minutes until a smooth mixture forms

Add the tapioca and allow it to sit for about 10 minutes

Bring the mixture to a boil over medium heat, making sure to keep stirring it from time to time

Pour the mix into serving dishes and enjoy!

Nutrition:

Calories: 51 Cal

Fats: 9 g

Carbs:13 g

Protein:2 g

266. Paper Thin Carrot Crisps

Preparation Time: 50 Minutes

Cooking Time: 10 Minute

Servings: 4

Ingredients:

3 cups of carrots sliced paper thin

2 tablespoon of olive oil

2 teaspoon of ground cumin

½ a teaspoon of smoked paprika

Pinch of salt

Directions:

Pre-heat your oven to 215-degree Fahrenheit

Slice up the carrots into paper thin coin shapes

Add the slices to a bowl and toss well with spices and oil

Mix and lay them out on a baking sheet lined up with parchment paper

Sprinkle salt

Bake for 8-10 minutes and enjoy!

Nutrition:

Calories: 280 Cal

Fat: 0 g

Carbs: 0 g

Protein: 0 g

267. Beautiful Mango and Chia Pudding

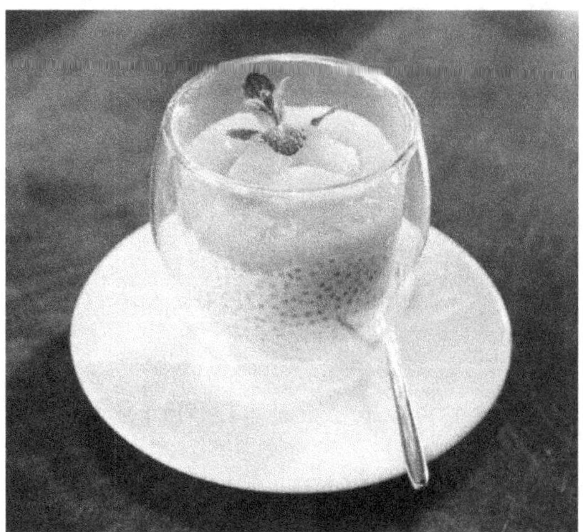

Preparation Time: 10 Minutes

Cooking Time: 60 Minutes

Servings: 4

Ingredients:

1 whole mango completely peeled up and pureed

1 whole cup of coconut milk

3 tablespoon of chia seed

Directions:

Take a bowl and add the listed ingredients

Give it a nice stir and allow them to chill for an hour. Serve!

Nutrition:

Calories: 146 Cal Fat: 26g Carbs: 15 g

Protein: 23 g

268. Sassy Chocolate Mousse

Preparation Time: 10 Minutes

Cooking Time: 0

Servings: 4

Ingredients:

Coconut cream scraped from the upper side of 2 pieces of 13.5-ounce chilled cans of full fat coconut milk

4 tablespoons of cocoa

3 tablespoons of Agave Nectar

1 teaspoon of vanilla extract

Directions:

Take a large bowl and scoop out the thick coconut cream from the can to the bowl

Add nectar, vanilla extract and cocoa to the bowl

Beat it well using an electric mixer, starting from low and going to medium until a foamy texture appears

Divide the mix evenly amongst ramekins and chill to your desired level of cold

Enjoy!

Nutrition:

Calories: 134 Cal

Fat: 3.8 g

Carbohydrates: 16 g

Protein: 3.8 g

269. Tender Heirloom Carrots

Preparation Time: 10 Minutes

Cooking Time: 45 Minute

Servings: 3-4

Ingredients: 1 bunch heirloom carrots

1 tablespoon of fresh thyme leaves

½ a tablespoon of coconut oil

1 tablespoon of maple syrup

1/8 cup of fresh squeeze orange juices

1/8 teaspoon of sea salt Salt as needed

Directions:

Pre-heat your oven to 350-degree Fahrenheit

Wash your carrots well and discard any green pieces

Take a small sized mixing bowl and add coconut oil, maple syrup, orange juice and a bit of salt

Pour the mixture over your carrots and spread on a large sized baking sheet

Sprinkle a bit of thyme and roast for 45 minutes

Sprinkle a generous amount of salt and a bit of thyme as garnish. Enjoy!

Nutrition:

Calories: 70 Cal Fat: 3 g Carbs: 11 g

Protein: 1 g

270. Salmon, Spinach & Kale Salad

Preparation Time: 10 Minutes

Cooking Time: 10 Minutes

Servings: 1

Ingredients:

For Salad:

¼ cup fresh orange juice

1 (4-ounce) salmon fillet

1 teaspoon raw honey

1½ cups fresh baby spinach

1 teaspoon coconut oil

1½ cups fresh baby kale

½ of avocado, peeled, pitted and sliced

1 orange, peeled, seeded and sectioned

3 tablespoons pomegranate seeds

For Dressing:

½ tablespoon coconut oil

1 teaspoon raw honey

2½ tablespoons fresh orange juice

Salt, to taste

Directions:

In a bowl, mix together ¼ cup of orange juice and salmon.

Refrigerate, covered for approximately a couple of hours.

Preheat the oven to 400 degrees F. Grease a tiny baking dish.

Coat each side of salmon fillet with honey evenly.

In a smaller frying pan, melt coconut oil on medium heat.

Add salmon fillet and cook for around 1-2 minutes per side.

Transfer the salmon fillet into prepared baking dish and bake for approximately 8-10 minutes.

Meanwhile in a substantial bowl, mix together all salad ingredients.

For dressing inside a microwave safe bowl, add coconut oil and homey and microwave for approximately 20 seconds or till melted.

Add orange juice and salt and beat well.

Pour dressing over salad and toss to coat well.

Top with salmon fillet and serve.

Nutrition:

Calories: 497 Cal Fat: 11 g

Carbs: 24 g Fiber: 12 g

Protein: 34 g

Conclusion

Here are a few tips and suggestions to keep in mind while making important changes to your diet and lifestyle:

•Try new foods and don't be afraid to taste something that's different, unique, or even unusual. Many exotic fruits and vegetables offer distinctive tastes, as well as health benefits that we may not be aware of. Mangos, guava, jackfruit, and seaweed are among some common and delicious options to try. Even some everyday foods that we pass by in the grocery store, such as avocado, aloe, lentils, and other foods that are nutritious and useful can be easily added to our everyday routine.

•Try a new recipe at least once a week, or if you're busy, once every two weeks. It doesn't have to be a complex option to impress guests, but merely a simple 3-4 ingredient dish that you enjoy. It will expand your palette and taste for new meals.

•Stay active and exercise often. Eating well is just one way to combat inflammation. Moving regularly and getting into a routine of exercise is beneficial. Studies indicate a positive impact on weight loss and health improvement from minimal exercise for 30 minutes each session for just three times a week. Walking regularly, cycling, and trying a variety of stretching and strength training exercises can help you develop muscle and tone while improving your health with diet.

•If you suffer from chronic conditions that trigger inflammation, do as much as possible to read and educate yourself on the symptoms, treatments, and what you can do to reduce the effects. Some conditions are difficult to cure, though many of the negative side effects and pain can be greatly reduced by improving diet, exercise, and everyday habits.

•If you smoke or drink excessive alcohol, it's in your best interest to quit both, or at least reduce your drinking significantly while reducing smoking. Since both habits can be difficult to tackle, there are resources available online to curb your cravings, and eating well is one way to improve your body's condition in the meantime.

If you feel discouraged after a while and experience an increase in symptoms associated with inflammation, it's best to check in with your doctor or a specialist to monitor your health and any related condition(s). Continue to eat healthily, and if you "cheat" now and again, just start again. Everyone makes mistakes and changing dietary habits can be challenging for anyone. Sometimes, there are experiences or circumstances in life that cause us to abandon our dietary plans, and this can make returning to this diet, as with any other way of eating, challenging. Always look forward and consider the benefits of following the diet previously, which can be inspiring to begin again.

www.ingramcontent.com/pod-product-compliance
Lightning Source LLC
Chambersburg PA
CBHW081950260726
48657CB00009BA/2522